Retinoblastoma - Past, Present and Future

Edited by Hind Manaa Alkatan

Published in London, United Kingdom

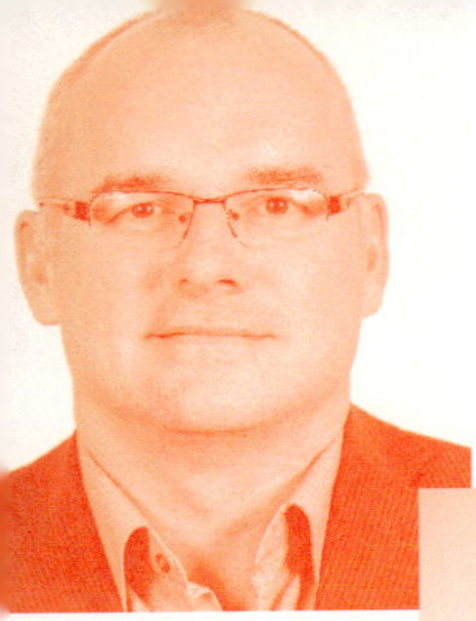
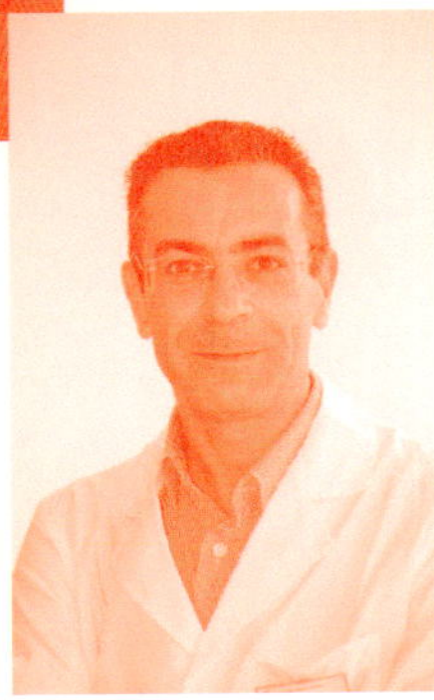
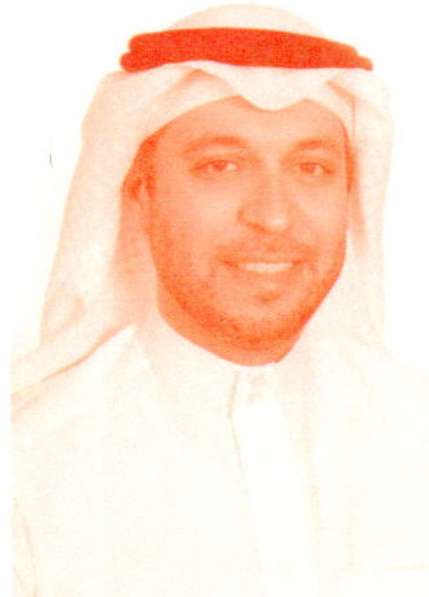
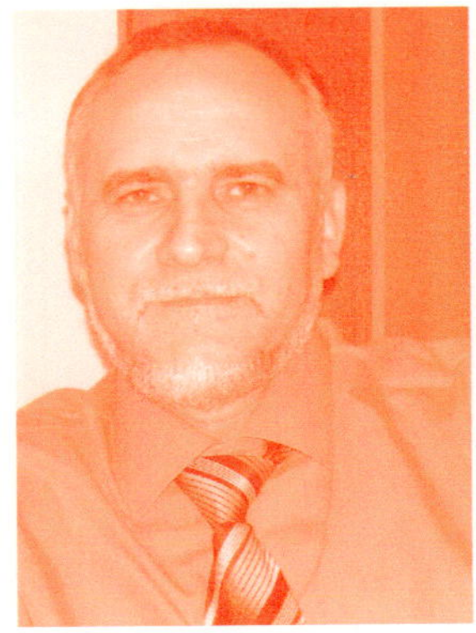
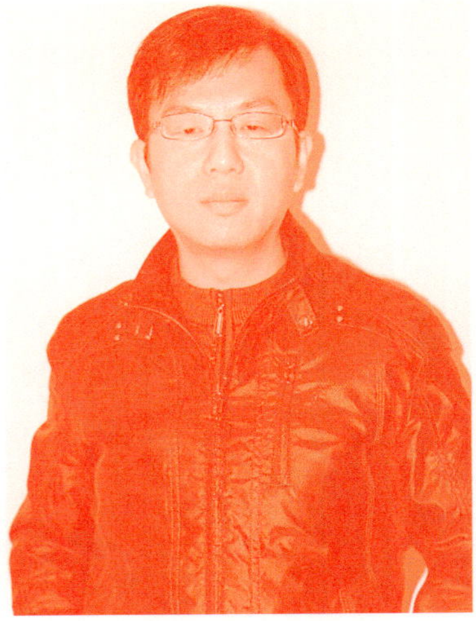
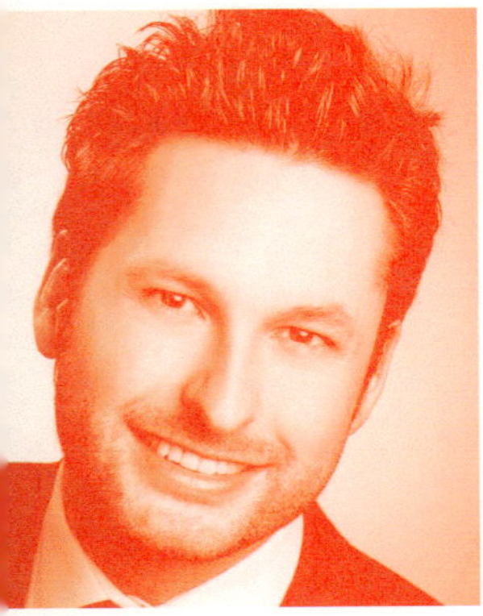
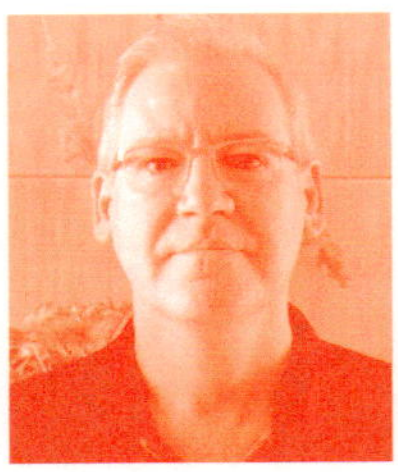

IntechOpen

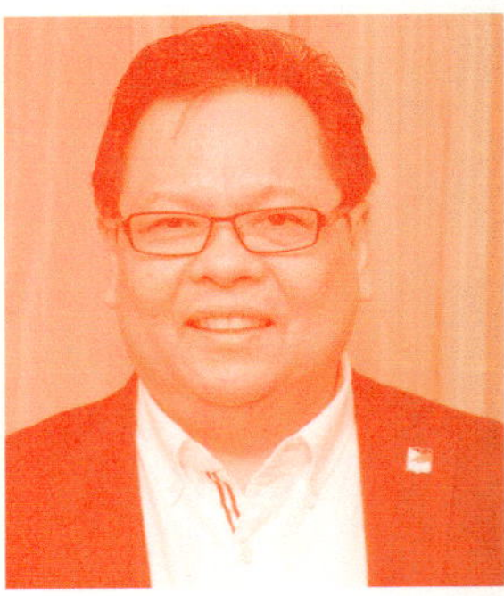
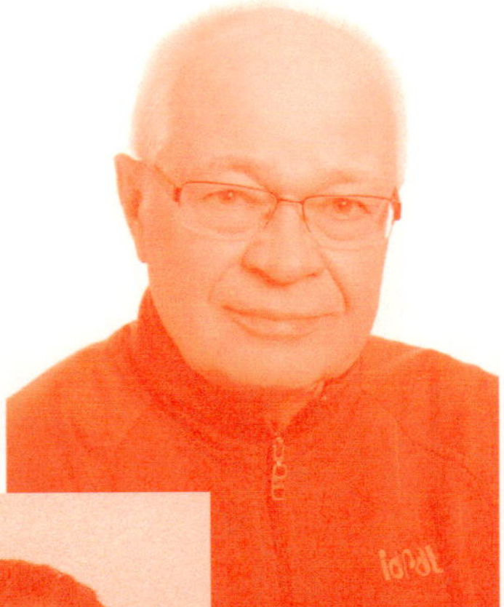
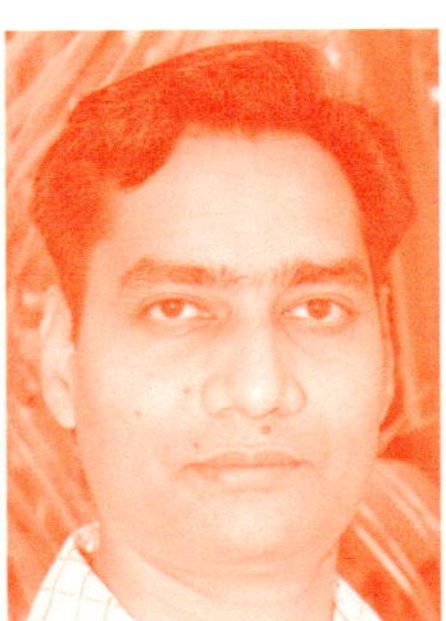
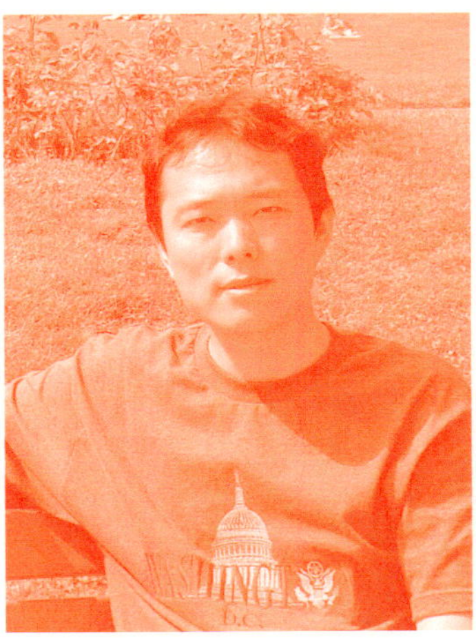
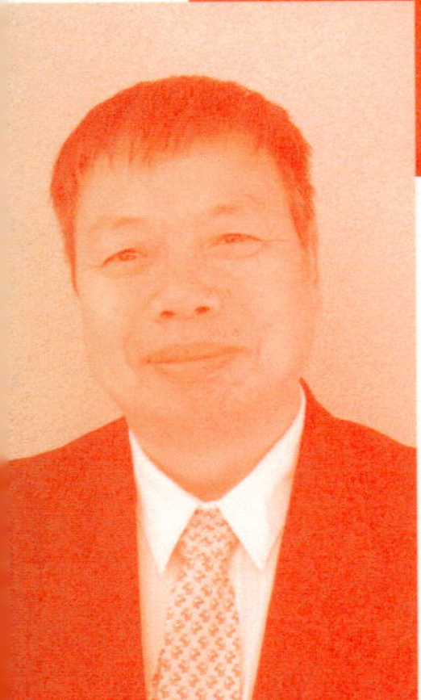
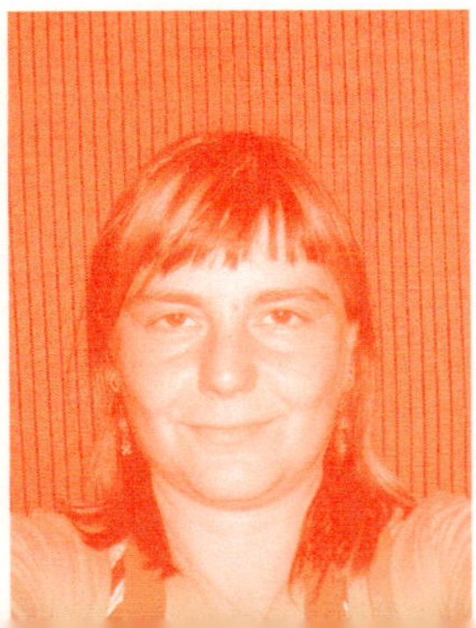

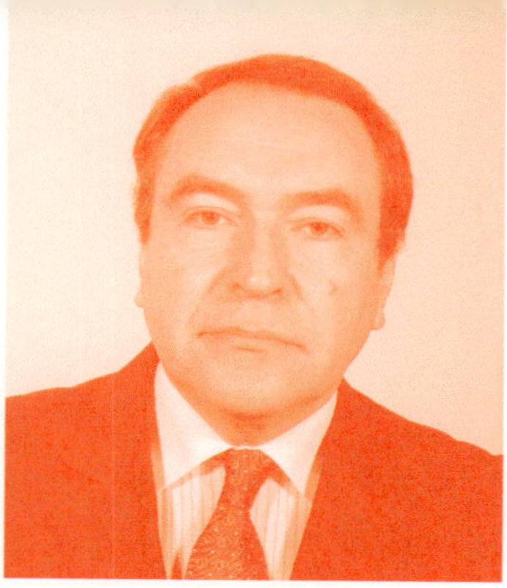
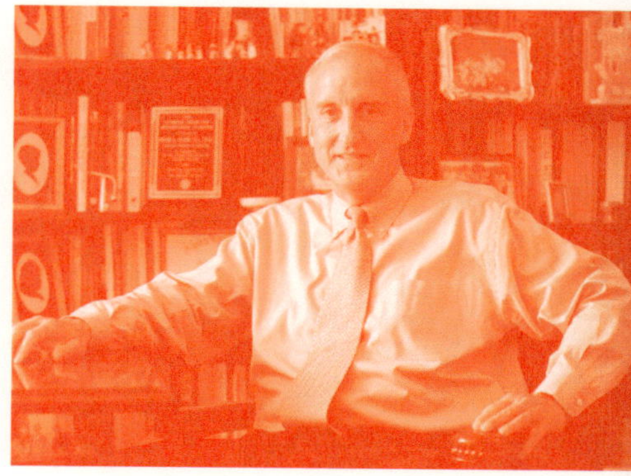
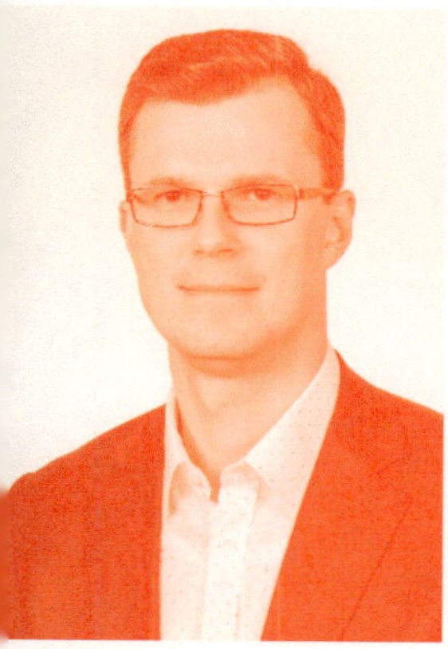
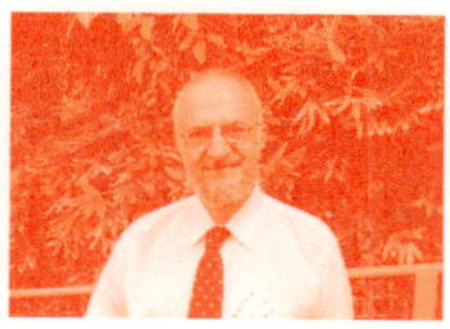
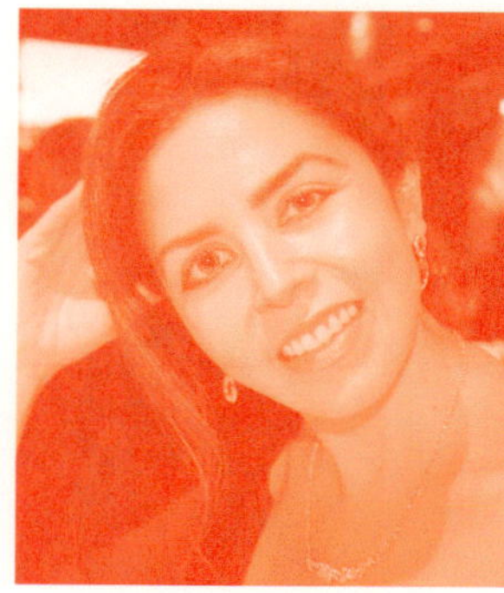

Supporting open minds since 2005

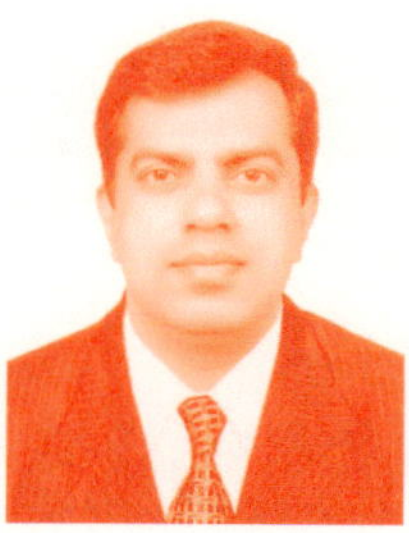
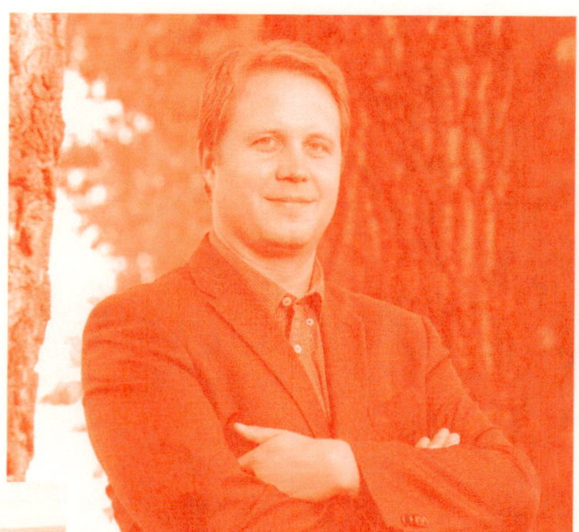
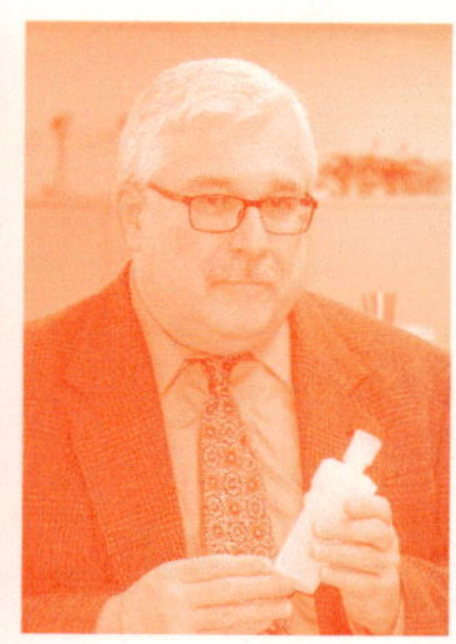
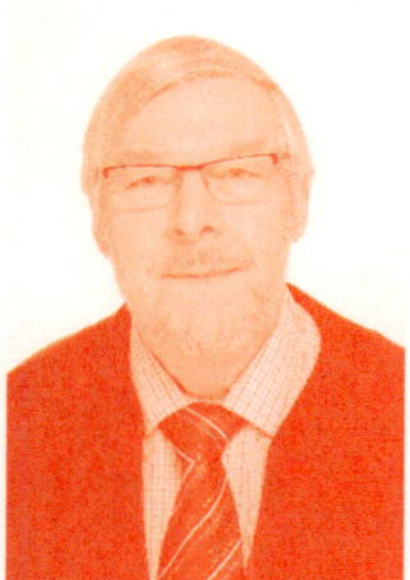
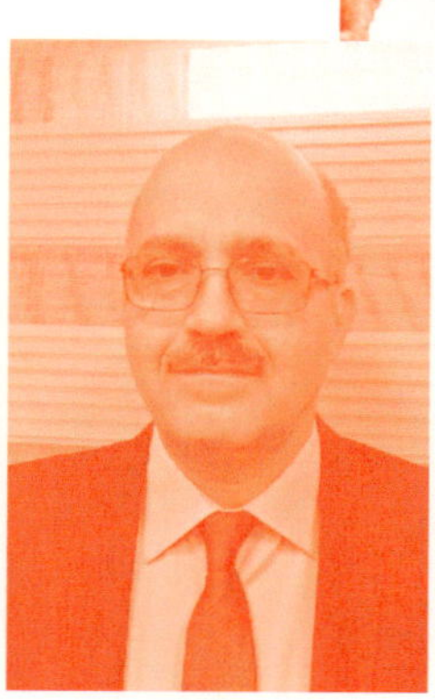
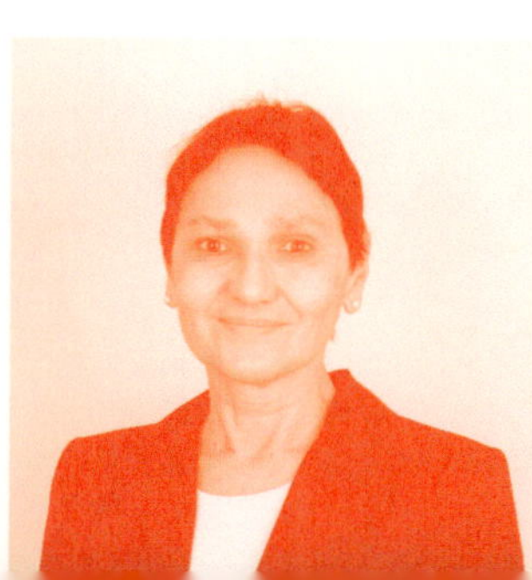
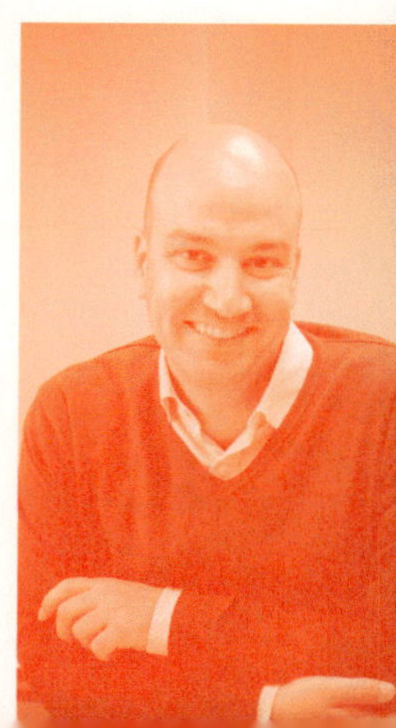

Retinoblastoma - Past, Present and Future
http://dx.doi.org/10.5772/intechopen.81455
Edited by Hind Manaa Alkatan

Contributors
Eman Al-Sharif, Amani Al Kofide, Azza Maktabi, Hala Helmi, Heba Alsharif, Spencer Langevin, Brian Marr, Tariq Al-Zahem, Abdullah Albahlal, Saad Aldahmash, Waleed Alsarhani, Leen Abu Safieh, Alena Furdova, Juraj Sekáč, Ido Didi Fabian, Dalal Fatani, Fahad Albader, Abdullah Almater, Saleh AlMesfer, Abdulrahman Alfaleh, Khalid Alshomar

First published in London, United Kingdom, 2019 by IntechOpen
IntechOpen is the global imprint of INTECHOPEN LIMITED, registered in England and Wales, registration number: 11086078, 7th floor, 10 Lower Thames Street, London, EC3R 6AF, United Kingdom
Printed in Croatia

British Library Cataloguing-in-Publication Data
A catalogue record for this book is available from the British Library

Additional hard and PDF copies can be obtained from orders@intechopen.com

Retinoblastoma - Past, Present and Future
Edited by Hind Manaa Alkatan
p. cm.
Print ISBN 978-1-78984-790-1
Online ISBN 978-1-78984-791-8
eBook (PDF) ISBN 978-1-83962-791-0

For EU product safety concerns:
IN TECH d.o.o., Prolaz Marije Krucifikse Kozulić 3, 51000 Rijeka, Croatia, info@intechopen.com or visit our website at intechopen.com.

Meet the editor

Dr. Hind Manaa Alkatan, MD, is Associate Professor, Consultant (Ophthalmology and Pathology), Chief of Ophthalmic Pathology, Director of the Post-Graduate Training Programs in Ophthalmology, and Associate Director for External Accreditation at Postgraduate Medical Education, King Saud University (KSU), Riyadh, Saudi Arabia. She obtained her Saudi Ophthalmology Board from KSU, and completed her postdoctoral studies in Oculoplastic, Pediatric Ophthalmology, and Ophthalmic Pathology from the University of Manitoba and the University of British Columbia, Canada. She is a member of international organizations: Eastern Ophthalmic Pathology, Canadian, and Saudi Ophthalmology Societies. She has been invited as a distinguished speaker to international symposia. She has published around 140 papers in reputed local and international journals and has been serving as an editorial board member for a number of other journals.

Contents

Preface

Retinoblastoma (RB) is the most common primary ocular malignancy of childhood. In the previous half century, universal treatment for this tumor has been limited to enucleation only. However, with evolving new treatment modalities, better understanding of the genetic background of this tumor with corresponding counseling, and improving health awareness, many specialized centers have been able to offer conservative management with preserved functional vision in many cases. The survival of affected children has also been dramatically improved.

This book is the product of collective unique information that covers all major aspects of this tumor starting from a description of the history of the disease. The first part of the book has been designed to take you on an interesting journey over history, including the distribution of RB throughout the world with epidemiological information and a brief genetic description. The second part extensively tackles the clinical presentation of the tumor highlighting the presence of late advanced cases in spite of increasing health awareness of this tumor. Then, within the same part of the book, readers will find a comprehensive summary of all treatment modalities used in the previous era of management, as well as the most recently updated therapeutic options. Diagnostic tools are also included in that part to show the value of radiological assessment and the importance of the histopathological careful evaluation of the tumor in enucleated globes. Classification of the tumor according to the American Joint Commission on Cancer is also described aiming to show its importance in the determination of further chemotherapy and as a guideline for prognosis. The last chapters in the second part also mention secondary malignancies and long-term follow-up in these patients.

The book is well written in a way that allows readers to grasp and retain the information, thus it is suitable as a baseline reference book for general ophthalmologists, residents under training, as well as highly specialized pediatric ophthalmologists/oncologists who are actually dealing with these patients. It is also of benefit to healthcare leaders who are interested in exploring the magnitude of the morbidity that is related to this tumor in children, especially in developing countries, to execute plans for health awareness and genetic counseling for a brighter future.

The collective information in this book comes from a wide range of sources with remarkable contributions from radiologists, pediatric oncologists, senior ophthalmologists who are directly involved in this field and who have much experience, and selected junior ophthalmologists. The editor would like to acknowledge all contributing authors.

Last but not least, the reader will find that the book is enjoyable and full of useful information with illustrations and images.

Dr. Hind Manaa Alkatan, MD
Associate Professor and Consultant,
Departments of Ophthalmology and Pathology,
Director of Postgraduate Residency and Fellowship Training Programs in Ophthalmology and Assistant Director for External Accreditation Unit,
Post-Graduate Medical Education Department,
Kind Saud University,
Riyadh, Saudi Arabia

Section 1

Basic Knowledge

Chapter 1

History and Genetics of Retinoblastoma

Tariq Alzahem, Waleed Alsarhani, Abdullah Albahlal, Leen Abu Safieh and Saad Aldahmash

Abstract

The history of retinoblastoma (RB) goes back to 1597 when Pieter Pawius of Amsterdam described a tumor that resembled retinoblastoma. "Fungus haematodes" was the first term used to describe retinoblastoma. Later, the American Ophthalmological Society approved the term retinoblastoma in 1926. The retinoblastoma protein is encoded by the RB1 gene located at 13q14. The functioning model of the tumor suppressor genes was first proposed by Alfred Knudson in the 1970s who precisely explained the hereditary mechanism of retinoblastoma. If both alleles of this gene are mutated, the protein is inactivated and this results in the development of retinoblastoma. One mutation can be either germline or somatic and the second one is always somatic. Differentiation between sporadic and germline retinoblastoma variants requires the identification of the RB1 germline status of the patient. This identification is important for assessing the risk of additional tumors in the same eye, the other eye, and the risk of secondary tumors. Thus, genetic testing is an important component of the management of all children diagnosed with retinoblastoma. In this chapter, we will go over the history, genetics, and counseling for patients with retinoblastoma.

Keywords: history, genetics, two-hit hypothesis, RB1 gene, tumor suppressor, epigenetics, Knudson, allele, germline, somatic

1. History

1.1 Introduction

Different tumors that resembled retinoblastoma were described in the past, the first of which was by Pieter Pawius of Amsterdam in 1597 [1]. The Dutch anatomist described a malignancy involving the left eye, temporal bone, and cranium [1]. Pawius described the tumor as "filled with substance like brain tissue mixed with thick blood and like crushed stone." The crushed stone may have represented retinoblastoma classic calcifications. Then, in 1767, Hayes described another case of a child who had presented with the appearance "cat's eyes in the dark" [2]. This was the first description of leukocoria in the scientific literature. In the last two centuries, retinoblastoma had different names. "Fungus haematodes" was the term used in the early 1800s. This term was used to describe a fungating vascular tumor that affected different parts of the body including the globe. Before the era of ophthalmoscopy, no one thought the tumor originated from the globe except

James Wardrop who had a different opinion. He believed "fungus haematodes" of the globe originated from the retina and should be recognized as a distinct entity [3]. Wardrop, who was a Scottish surgeon, reached this conclusion based on his dissections. However, at that time, Wardrop's explanation and observation were not acknowledged. Wardrop was also the first surgeon to perform enucleation for retinoblastoma [3]. In 1854, Virchow suggested the term "glioma of the retina" [4]. Flexner and later Wintersteiner noticed tumor rosettes on histopathology which resembled the photoreceptors of the retina [5, 6]. Flexner proposed the name neuroepithelioma, and both thought that the photoreceptors were the origin of the tumor [5]. Finally, in 1922, Verhoeff coined the term retinoblastoma after he noticed the histologic similitude between the disease and embryonic retina [7]. Four years later, the American Ophthalmological Society decided to adopt the term retinoblastoma. In 1970, Tso described the appearance of fleurettes which represent advanced photoreceptor differentiation [8].

1.2 Retinoblastoma variants

Hirschberg categorized the disease per its growth into endophytum and exophytum [9]. In 1960, Schofield described few cases who had presented with hypopyon and no macroscopic evidence of retinoblastoma [10]. After enucleation, histological exam showed malignant cells and rosettes were found within the retina. He described the cases as having "diffuse infiltrating retinoblastoma" [10]. He gave the credit to Ashton who first used the term in 1958 after personal communication with him. Schofield stressed on including retinoblastoma as part of the differential diagnosis of hypopyon. In 1998, Grossniklaus was the first to use the name "anterior variant of diffuse retinoblastoma" [11]. He reported a case that was misdiagnosed as anterior uveitis. After the eye was enucleated, the tumor was found to be in the peripheral retina, iris, ciliary body, and anterior vitreous. In 1982, Bader et al. described three cases of trilateral retinoblastoma [12]. He found out retinoblastoma-like tumors in the suprasellar or parasellar region few months before the detection of intraocular retinoblastoma in each of the three cases. He concluded the association was more than a coincidence and having retinoblastoma gene may confer the risk of having other "ectopic" malignancies.

1.3 The history of genetics

In the 1800s, retinoblastoma was thought to be an autosomal dominant hereditary disease. Alfred Knudson, a cancer geneticist, had observed that patients with hereditary retinoblastoma developed multiple tumors in both eyes, while patients with the non-hereditary form had unilateral tumors. In 1971, Knudson proposed the two-hit hypothesis. It states that a second sporadic mutation should occur in patients with hereditary retinoblastoma before the development of retinoblastoma [13]. The other type described by Knudson was non-hereditary retinoblastoma. In non-hereditary retinoblastoma, two sporadic mutations in both alleles of retinal cells should take place. In 1986, RB gene was the first tumor suppressor gene to be identified in medical history.

1.4 The treatment history

Wardrop advocated enucleation in 1809 as the only treatment [3]. However, Wardrop's patients failed to survive despite enucleation. Von Graefe suggested the optic nerve should be excised during enucleation. This resulted in better survival rates. One of the major turn points in the history of retinoblastoma was introduction of ophthalmoscope, which allowed earlier detection of retinoblastoma. Retinoblastoma was a fatal disease, so the primary was aim to save life of affected patients. The first radiation treatment for retinoblastoma was reported, in 1903, by Hilgartner in Texas [14]. Hilgartner reported the survival of the patient but not the eye following a series of X-rays. Verhoeff, in 1921, used radiotherapy to cure retinoblastoma [15]. However, 60 years following radiation therapy, Verhoeff's patient developed lid basal cell carcinoma and recurrence of retinoblastoma [16]. In 1930, Moore used surgically inserted radioactive radon seed to cure retinoblastoma [17]. Weve introduced the use of diathermy for treating retinoblastoma [18]. However, it resulted in major complications including large chorioretinal scarring and scleral thinning. Then, Stallard established plaque brachytherapy [19]. External beam radiotherapy (EBRT) was used and resulted in improvement in eye survival rates [20]. However, EBRT cause second cancers in patients with germline mutations by causing the second hit described by Knudson [21, 22].

Schwickerath used xenon arc photocoagulation to treat retinoblastoma [23]. Harvey Lincoff developed cryotherapy for the treatment of small retinoblastoma tumors [24]. In 1953, Kupfer was the first to use chemotherapy, nitrogen mustard, along with radiotherapy for retinoblastoma [25]. To decrease systemic side effects of chemotherapy, the idea of local chemotherapy came up. Kaneko used intra-arterial chemotherapy for retinoblastoma, which resulted in substantially higher drug concentration in the eye [26, 27]. Retinoblastoma mortality rate decreased substantially from 100 to 2% in the last 50 years [25]. Indeed, retinoblastoma is a story of success and there is still more to come.

2. Genetics of retinoblastoma

2.1 Introduction

Retinoblastoma (RB) is the most common intraocular malignancy in children affecting 1 in 18,000 live births which occurs as a result of biallelic inactivation of RB1 gene [28]. Hereditary RB is due to heterozygous germline mutation in one copy of the RB1 gene, hence is inherited as an autosomal dominant trait. In this form, all body cells have a dysfunctional RB1 allele and, thus, are vulnerable to neoplasia. The non-hereditary form of RB is consequent to somatic mutations, which is known to affect both RB1 alleles in retinal cells [29].

In these patients, RB development requires a second, somatic, mutation in the same cells that renders the other allele nonfunctional. The cumulative incidence rates of non-ocular tumors reach up to 90% at 30 years in patients who were exposed to radiation vs. 68% at 32 years in patients without radiation exposure [30].

The aim of this chapter is to provide a valuable summary of retinoblastoma genetics that is essential for genetic counseling and estimation of short-term (multifocal and bilateral ocular tumors) and long-term (secondary tumors) risks with an overall improvement of healthcare planning and management of our patients.

2.2 The RB1 gene and protein function

The RB1 gene located on the long arm of chromosome 13 (13q14) is a negative regulator element in the cell cycle process and was the first tumor suppressor gene identified [31]. This gene codes for the RB protein which has multiple cellular functions; it prevents the dividing cells from uncontrollable cycles in the mitosis stage and has a role in genomic stability, apoptosis, and differentiation [32]. Inactivation of the RB protein is usually caused by deletions and nonsense mutations [33].

2.3 Inheritance of retinoblastoma

Retinoblastoma is an autosomal dominant inherited disease. Thus, there is a 50% risk of inheriting a germline mutation for each child born to a patient with a germline RB1 mutation. However, 90% of the children with a germline RB1 mutation will develop retinoblastoma with an overall risk of having a child with hereditary retinoblastoma of 45%. The remaining 10% of children with the mutated RB1 gene will be unaffected carriers [34].

More than 900 mutations have been identified in the RB1gene. Different types of mutations have been identified in RB1 gene; deletions and gene rearrangements represent majority of mutations (http://www.hgmd.cf.ac.uk/ac/gene.php?gene=RB1). Additionally, de novo mutation is considered to be present in most children with heritable retinoblastoma, as a positive family history is elicited in only 10% of all affected children, which is then transmissible in subsequent generations. In these children, in whom a germline mutation is present with a negative family history, 30% have bilateral disease and 60% develop unilateral RB [35]. A germline RB1 mutation is present in 15% of children diagnosed with a unilateral RB [34].

The "2-hit" hypothesis, which was first proposed by Knudson, described two complementary mutations that are essential for the development of hereditary and non-hereditary forms of retinoblastoma. The first "hit," or mutation, in heritable retinoblastoma is a germline mutation affecting all body cells. The second mutation is a somatic mutation occurring in many retinoblasts with subsequent multifocal or bilateral lesion. On the other hand, the first and second mutations in non-heritable retinoblastoma occur somatically in a single retinoblast presenting as a unilateral and unifocal retinoblastoma [36].

2.4 Epigenetics of RB

Epigenetics is the study of heritable changes occurring in gene activity and expression of a specific phenotype. These changes do not cause alterations in the DNA sequence, external and/or environmental factors might affect cellular and physiological phenotypic traits [37].

RB1 gene has been linked to the regulation of numerous epigenetic processes. These processes include DNA methylation, histone modification, and microRNA regulation [38–43]. In addition, dysfunction of RB1 gene causes deregulations in many tumor suppressor pathways. Tumorigenesis requires this epigenetic deregulation against which new therapeutic options can be invented. Retinoblastoma was the first tumor discovered to be showing the actions of epigenetics on the pathogenesis of cancer [44].

2.4.1 MicroRNAs in RB

MicroRNAs are small, conserved, single-stranded, and non-coding RNA that comprise 1–5% of the human genome and are involved in regulating at least 30% of protein-coding genes [45–49]. MicroRNAs play an essential role in the regulation of gene expression governing various cellular and metabolic pathways [50–56]. MicroRNAs' deregulation has been linked to the development of RB and other human diseases [57–59]. Thus, microRNA studies on RB have offered novel understandings of the disease mechanisms. Messenger RNA (mRNA), a large family of RNA molecules that convey genetic information from DNA to ribosome, was also studied in cases of RB. A three-fold increase was noted in mRNA levels of ACVR1C/ALK7 in retinoblastomas invading the optic nerve. This suggests that ACVR1C/SMAD2 pathway has a function in promoting invasion and growth of RB [60].

2.4.2 DNA methylation

DNA methylation involves the addition of methyl groups to the DNA molecule. This process can change the DNA segment activity without altering its sequence. When this segment is located in a gene promoter, DNA methylation usually acts to block gene transcription. The role for promoter methylation in retinoblastoma development was discovered when there was methylation of a CpG island (CpG 106) that overlapped the RB1 promoter [61]. This has resulted in a decreased gene expression confirming the epigenetic factor in retinoblastoma tumorigenesis [44, 62–64].

Methylation of DNA segment was also reported in tumor suppressor genes beyond RB1. These genes include RASSF1A (RAS-associated domain family 1A) that was methylated in 59% of tumors analyzed and adenomatous polyposis coli (APC) in 6% [65]. Furthermore, hypermethylation of O6-methylguanine-DNA methyltransferase (MGMT) was detected in 15% of RB tumors. This was associated with advanced-stage RB suggesting that the presence of methylated MGMT is a poor prognostic indicator [66].

2.5 Features of heritable RB

2.5.1 13q deletion syndrome

Children with this syndrome may present with characteristic dysmorphic features, developmental delay, and intellectual disability. Interstitial chromosome deletion or translocation of region 13q14 was found in approximately 6% of patients with RB [67]. The larger the size of chromosomal deletion, the more severe the associations. Dysmorphic facial features include high and broad forehead, short nose, prominent philtrum, and a thick everted lower lip [67]. Karyotype or chromosomal microarray is usually performed to detect chromosomal deletions, translocations, and copy number alteration [68].

2.5.2 Trilateral RB

Trilateral retinoblastoma indicates the concomitant presence of a heritable retinoblastoma and a midline tumor or a pineoblastoma [12, 69]. Around 5–13% of patients with RB develop trilateral retinoblastoma [70]. Therefore, in children with heritable retinoblastoma, a brain magnetic resonance imaging with gadolinium contrast every 6 months is recommended until the age of 5 years [71].

2.5.3 Secondary malignant neoplasms

As patients with heritable RB age, the risk of non-ocular malignancies significantly increases. These tumors include osteosarcoma, soft tissue sarcoma, epithelial cancers, and melanoma. It has been suggested that a greater risk for second cancers occurs in patients with familial RB compared with those with a de novo RB1 mutation [72]. External beam radiation therapy for patients with heritable disease has a further increased risk of developing second malignancies.

2.5.4 Low-penetrant retinoblastoma

In a typical "null" germline mutation, there is a 90% chance that patient will develop RB. In a few families, however, the penetrance is far less than 90% with subsequent reduced expressivity and an increased proportion of unilateral RB. Some patients will be carriers with no tumors [73]. These low-penetrant mutations are usually missense mutations. Moreover, a low level of RB protein production due to mutations in the promoter region can occur without total absence of the protein [33].

2.6 Genetic testing

2.6.1 Clinical context

Heritability of retinoblastoma is confirmed if a proband with retinoblastoma has a family history of retinoblastoma. In the absence of family history of RB, genetic testing is required to identify heterozygous germline RB1 pathogenic variants. This will allow early diagnosis and identification of potential carriers of the heritable RB1 mutations which eventually will improve disease management and family counseling.

The following staging system has been proposed to facilitate description of one's genetic risk of possessing germline RB1 pathogenic variant: [74, 75]

HX	Unknown or insufficient evidence of a constitutional (germline) RB1 pathogenic variant
H0	Normal RB1 alleles in blood tested with demonstrated high-sensitivity assays
H0*	Normal RB1 in blood with <1% residual risk for mosaicism
H1	Bilateral retinoblastoma, trilateral retinoblastoma (retinoblastoma with intracranial CNS midline embryonic tumor), family history of retinoblastoma, or RB1 pathogenic variant identified in blood

2.6.2 Single-gene testing

For bilateral, unilateral familial, and unilateral multifocal retinoblastoma, peripheral blood DNA should be tested initially using sequence analysis and gene-targeted deletion/duplication analysis of RB1. If blood testing did not reveal any mutation, molecular analysis of tumor DNA (if either eye was enucleated) should subsequently be done. Mosaicism can be assumed if germline mutation was not found in this group of patients [76].

For unilateral unifocal non-familial retinoblastoma, the chance of carrying RB1 germline mutation is 15%. And, with the high sensitivity of RB1 mutation detection techniques which reach up to (95%), testing blood from unilateral patients, extracted at the time of the first examination under anesthesia may confirm the diagnosis of germline RB1 mutation. If blood DNA testing did not reveal any mutation, molecular analysis of tumor DNA (if the eye was enucleated) should subsequently be done. If pathogenic variants were detected in the tissue, the blood DNA should be re-tested looking for these specific variants or any large rearrangements within the RB1 gene. If tumor tissue was unavailable, a negative blood result will reduce the chance of possessing a mutation to less than 1%. With such very low risk of RB development, the proband needs no additional exam under anesthesia and frequent examination in the clinic is sufficient. The same conclusion also applies to the offspring.

It has been previously reported by Rushlow et al. that retinoblastoma is not exclusively caused by mutations in RB1 gene; mutations in MYCN oncogene has been predicted to be responsible for 18% of cases diagnosed with non-familial unilateral RB in children less than 6 months of age. They reported group of patients who harbored mutations in MYCN amplification and no RB1 mutations. An additional 1.5% of patients with unilateral non-familial RB were found to have normal RB1 and MYCN genes [77].

2.6.3 Chromosomal microarray (CMA)

Chromosomal microarray analysis (CMA) is a technology used for the detection of clinically significant microdeletions or duplications and genetic rearrangement (including RB1), with a high sensitivity for submicroscopic aberrations [78]. It can be utilized in retinoblastoma patients with dysmorphic features, developmental delay, and/or other congenital anomalies [79, 80].

2.7 Genetic counseling

Genetic testing and counseling are essential parts of RB disease management; they help delineate heritable RB for non-heritable ones. The increased knowledge of molecular basis of RB allowed for better understanding and management of the disease. Genetic evaluation and counseling should be done in collaboration with a geneticist and genetic counselor [81]. The aim of the geneticist is to implement the proper test to detect the underlying disease causing mutation and communicate with the genetic counselor who will educate patients and their families about their condition in general, discuss anticipated risk of developing subsequent tumors, and construct the appropriate screening plan for the affected individual and their relatives.

At first encounter of a patient and family of retinoblastoma, detailed family history should be obtained and family pedigree should be drawn with special attention to relatives at risk. Then, genetic testing is offered after discussion about purpose, possible outcome, and limitations. Specimens are then collected and sent to a specialized laboratory for analysis. Another counseling session is arranged to convey and interpret the reported results. Accordingly, additional testing and counseling should be offered to the relatives at risk.

2.7.1 Prenatal screening

In the presence of family history of retinoblastoma and when a specific RB1 mutation is detected, a pregnancy at risk can be tested by chorionic villus sampling or amniocentesis. Prenatal testing and preimplantation genetic diagnosis are indicated as approximately 30% of newborns with an RB1 mutation will harbor a vision-threatening tumor [82, 83].

Amniocentesis can be used to screen the fetus for carrying *RB1* gene using the above-mentioned methods. If an *RB1* pathogenic variant was identified, then fetal ultrasonography may be used to identify intraocular tumor as small as 2–3 mm in size [84]. If tumors are present, preterm delivery to allow early treatment may be indicated. Alternatively, early term delivery (i.e., 36–38 weeks gestation) can be induced even if no intraocular tumor can be detected as this was found to improve the visual outcome and reduce the need for invasive tests and therapies in the postnatal period [83, 85].

Prenatal testing and management may raise several ethical issues especially if it involved termination of pregnancy. A generally accepted approach is to discuss all options with the parents and leave them to decide on further steps.

2.7.2 Genetic screening and counseling after birth

Genetic testing should be performed carefully especially when the propand's blood is found negative for pathogenic mutations. It remains possible that large genetic rearrangement is being missed or they are mosaicism for RB1 mutation.

Carriers of RB1 pathogenic variants should be frequently examined for development of new tumors whether under anesthesia or in the outpatient setting until they reach 9 years of age and the frequency of follow-ups should be reduced thereafter. For relatives who do not carry the mutation, no additional monitoring is required [86]. However, proband's offspring will always be at risk of developing RB and be tested for the RB1 pathogenic mutation identified and proper counseling and clinical monitoring should be implemented. Additionally, all retinoblastoma survivors should have life-long surveillance for other lethal secondary tumors [21, 87, 88].

Conflict of interest

We do not have any financial interest to declare.

Author details

Tariq Alzahem[1*], Waleed Alsarhani[1], Abdullah Albahlal[2], Leen Abu Safieh[3] and Saad Aldahmash[1]

1 King Saud University, Riyadh, Saudi Arabia

2 King Khaled Eye Specialist Hospital, Riyadh, Saudi Arabia

3 King Fahad Medical City, Riyadh, Saudi Arabia

*Address all correspondence to: t.alzahem@hotmail.com

References

[1] Pawius P. Observatio XXIII. Tumor oculorum. In: Observationes Anatomicae Selectiores Appended to: Bartholinus T. Historiarum Anatomicarum Rariorum, Centuria III & IV. Copenhagen: Denmark Petrus Morsing; 1657

[2] Hayes R. The Case of a diseased eye communicated to Mr. William Hunter by Mr. Hayes, Surgeon. In: Medical Observations and Inquiries. By a Society of Physicans in London. Vol. 3. London: William Johnston; 1767. p. 120

[3] Wardrop J. Observations on the Fungus Haematodes or Soft Cancer. Edinburgh: George Ramsay and Co; 2013. p. 1809

[4] Virchow R. Die Krankehaften Geschwulste. Vol. Vol. 2. Berlin: August Hirshwald; 1864. pp. 151-169

[5] Flexner S. A peculiar glioma (neuroepithelioma?) of the retina. Bulletin of the Johns Hopkins Hospital. 1891;**2**:115-119

[6] Wintersteiner H. Das Neuroepithelioma Retinae. Eine Anatomische Und Klinische Studie. Vienna: Franz Deuticke; 1897

[7] Verhoeff FH, Jackson E. Minutes of the proceedings, 62nd annual meeting. Transactions of the American Ophthalmological Society. 1926;**24**:38-43

[8] Tso MOM, Zimmerman LE, Fine BS. The nature of retinoblastoma: I. photoreceptor differentiation. A clinical and histopathologic study. American Journal of Ophthalmology. 1970;**69**:339-349

[9] Hirschberg J. Die Markschwann die Natzhaut. Berlin: Hirschwald; 1869

[10] Schofield PB. Diffuse infiltrating retinoblastoma. The British Journal of Ophthalmology. 1960;**44**:35-41

[11] Grossniklaus HE, Dhaliwal RS, Martin DF. Diffuse anterior retinoblastoma. Retina. 1998;**18**(3):238-241

[12] Bader JL, Meadows AT, Zimmerman LE, Rorke LB, Voute PA, Champion LA, et al. Bilateral retinoblastoma with ectopic intracranial retinoblastoma: Trilateral retinoblastoma. Cancer Genetics and Cytogenetics. 1982;**5**(3):203-213

[13] Knudson AG Jr. Mutation and cancer: A statistical study of retinoblas Toma. Proceedings of the National Academy of Sciences of the United States of America. 1971;**68**:820-823

[14] Hilgartner HL. Report of a case of double glioma treated by x-ray. Texas Med Journal. 1903;**18**:322-332

[15] Verhoeff FH. Retinoblastoma successfully treated with x-rays: Normal vision retained after thirty-four years. Second report on a case. Archives of Ophthalmology. 1952;**48**:720-722

[16] Albert DM, McGhee CNJ, Seddon JM, Weichselbaum RR. Development of additional primary tumors after 62 years in the first patient with retinoblastoma cured by radiation therapy. American Journal of Ophthalmology. 1984;**97**:189-196

[17] Moore RF, Stallard HB, Milner JG. Retinal gliomata treated by radon seeds. The British Journal of Ophthalmology. 1931;**15**:673-696

[18] Weve HJM. On diathermy in ophthalmic practice. Transactions of the Ophthalmological Societies of the United Kingdom. 1939;**15**:43-80

[19] Stallard HB. The treatment of retinoblastoma. Ophthalmologica. 1966;**151**:214-230

[20] Reese AB, Ellsworth RM. The evaluation and current concept of retinoblastoma therapy. Transactions - American Academy of Ophthalmology and Otolaryngology. 1963;**67**:164-172

[21] Fletcher O, Easton D, Anderson K, Gilham C, Jay M, Peto J. Lifetime risks of common cancers among retinoblastoma survivors. Journal of the National Cancer Institute. 2004;**96**:357-363

[22] Kleinerman RA, Tucker MA, Tarone RE, Abramson DH, Seddon JM, Stovall M, et al. Risk of new cancers after radiotherapy in long-term survivors of retinoblastoma: An extended follow-up. Journal of Clinical Oncology. 2005;**23**:2272-2279

[23] Meyer-Schwickerath G. Lichtkoagulation. Albrecht von Graefe's Archiv für Ophthalmologie. 1954;**156**:2-34

[24] Lincoff H, McLean J, Long R. The cryosurgical treatment of intraocular tumors. American Journal of Ophthalmology. 1967;**63**:389-399

[25] MacCarthy A, Birch JM, Draper GJ, Hungerford JL, Kingston JE, Kroll ME, et al. Retinoblastoma: Treatment and survival in Great Britain 1963 to 2002. The British Journal of Ophthalmology. 2009;**93**:38-39

[26] Yamane T, Kaneko A, Mohri M. The technique of ophthalmic arterial infusion therapy for patients with intraocular retinoblastoma. International Journal of Clinical Oncology. 2004;**9**:69-73

[27] Taich P, Requejo F, Asprea M, Sgroi M, Gobin P, Abramson DH, et al. Topotecan delivery to the optic nerve after ophthalmic artery chemosurgery. PLoS One. 2016;**11**:e0151343

[28] Kivela T. The epidemiological challenge of the most frequent eye cancer: Retinoblastoma, an issue of birth and death. The British Journal of Ophthalmology. 2009;**93**:1129-1131

[29] Lee V, Hungerford JL, Bunce C, Ahmed F, Kingston JE, Plowman PN. Globe conserving treatment of the only eye in bilateral retinoblastoma. The British Journal of Ophthalmology. 2003;**87**:1374-1380

[30] Abramson DH, Ellsworth RM, Kitchin FD, Tung G. Second nonocular tumors in retinoblastoma survivors. Are they radiation-induced? Ophthalmology. 1984;**91**:1351-1355

[31] Hong FD, Huang HJ, To H, et al. Structure of the human retinoblastoma gene. Proceedings of the National Academy of Sciences of the United States of America. 1989;**86**:5502-5506

[32] Korenjak M, Anderssen E, Ramaswamy S, et al. RBF binding to both canonical E2F targets and noncanonical targets depends on functional dE2F/dDP complexes. Molecular and Cellular Biology. 2012;**32**:4375-4387

[33] Valverde JR, Alonso J, Palacios I, et al. *RB1 gene* mutation up-date, a meta-analysis based on 932 reported mutations available in a searchable database. BMC Genetics. 2005;**6**:53

[34] Gallie B, Erraguntla V, Heon E, et al. Retinoblastoma. In: Taylor D, Hoyt C, editors. Pediatric Ophthalmology and Strabismus. 3rd ed. London: Elsevier; 2004. pp. 486-504

[35] Draper GJ, Sanders BM, Brownbill PA, et al. Patterns of risk of hereditary retinoblastoma and applications to genetic counselling. British Journal of Cancer. 1992;**66**:211-219

[36] Knudson AG Jr. Mutation and cancer: Statistical study of retinoblastoma. Proceedings of the National Academy of Sciences of the United States of America. 1971;**68**:820-823

[37] Dupont C, Armant DR, Brenner CA. Epigenetics: Definition, mechanisms and clinical perspective. Seminars in Reproductive Medicine. 2009;**27**(5):351-357

[38] Chi P, Allis CD, Wang GG. Covalent histone modifications—Miswritten, misinterpreted and mis-erased in human cancers. Nature Reviews. Cancer. 2010;**10**:457-469

[39] Lu J, Ruhf M-L, Perrimon N, Leder P. A genome wideRNA interferencescreenidentifiesputative chromatin regulators essential for E2F repression. Proceedings of the National Academy of Sciences of the United States of America. 2007;**104**:9381-9386

[40] Benetti R, Gonzalo S, Jaco I, Muñoz P, Gonzalez S, et al. A mammalian microRNA cluster controls DNA methylation and telomere recombination via Rbl2-dependent regulation of DNA methyltrans- ferases. Nature Structural & Molecular Biology. 2008;**15**:998

[41] Wen H, Andrejka L, Ashton J, Karess R, Lipsick JS. Epigenetic regulation of gene expression by Drosophila Myb and E2F2-RBF via the Myb-MuvB/dREAM complex. Genes & Development. 2008;**22**:601-614

[42] Bourgo RJ, Siddiqui H, Fox S, Solomon D, Sansam CG, et al. SWI/SNF deficiency results in aberrant chromatin organization, mitotic failure, and diminished proliferative capacity. Molecular Biology of the Cell. 2009;**20**:3192-3199

[43] Gonzalo S, Blasco MA. Role of Rb family in the epigenetic definition of chromatin. Cell Cycle. 2005;**4**:752-755

[44] Zhang J, Benavente CA, McEvoy J, Flores-Otero J, Ding L, et al. A novel retinoblastoma therapy from genomic and epigenetic analyses. Nature. 2012;**481**:329-334

[45] Rajewsky N. L(ou)sy miRNA targets? Nature Structural & Molecular Biology. 2006;**13**:754-755

[46] Rajewsky N. microRNA target predictions in animals. Nature Genetics. 2006;**38**(Suppl):S8-S13

[47] Liu W, Mao SY, Zhu WY. Impact of tiny miRNAs on cancers. World Journal of Gastroenterology. 2007;**13**:497-502

[48] Berezikov E, Guryev V, van de Belt J, Wienholds E, Plasterk RH, Cuppen E. Phylogenetic shadowing and computational identification of human microRNA genes. Cell. 2005;**120**:21-24

[49] Stanczyk J, Pedrioli DM, Brentano F, Sanchez-Pernaute O, Kolling C, Gay RE, et al. Altered expression of MicroRNA in synovial fibroblasts and synovial tissue in rheumatoid arthritis. Arthritis and Rheumatism. 2008;**58**:1001-1009

[50] Esau C, Davis S, Murray SF, Yu XX, Pandey SK, Pear M, et al. miR-122 regulation of lipid metabolism revealed by *in vivo* antisense targeting. Cell Metabolism. 2006;**3**:87-98

[51] Krutzfeldt J, Rajewsky N, Braich R, Rajeev KG, Tuschl T, Manoharan M, et al. Silencing of microRNAs *in vivo* with 'antagomirs'. Nature. 2005;**438**:685-689

[52] Zhao Y, Samal E, Srivastava D. Serum response factor regulates a muscle-specific microRNA that targets Hand2 during cardiogenesis. Nature. 2005;**436**:214-220

[53] Naguibneva I, Ameyar-Zazoua M, Polesskaya A, Ait-Si-Ali S, Groisman R, Souidi M, et al. The microRNA miR-181 targets the homeobox protein Hox-A11 during mammalian myoblast differentiation. Nature Cell Biology. 2006;**8**:278-284

[54] Garzon R, Pichiorri F, Palumbo T, Iuliano R, Cimmino A, Aqeilan R, et al. MicroRNA fingerprints during human

mega-karyocytopoiesis. Proceedings of the National Academy of Sciences of the United States of America. 2006;**103**:5078-5083

[55] Monticelli S, Ansel KM, Xiao C, Socci ND, Krichevsky AM, Thai TH, et al. MicroRNA profiling of the murine hematopoietic system. Genome Biology. 2005;**6**:R71

[56] Ambros V. The functions of animal microRNAs. Nature. 2004;**431**:350-355

[57] Li BQ, Zhang J, Huang T, Zhang L, Cai YD. Identification of retinoblastoma related genes with shortest path in a protein-protein interaction network. Biochimie. 2012;**94**:1910-1917

[58] Dalgard CL, Gonzalez M, deNiro JE, O'Brien JM. Differential microRNA-34a expression and tumor suppressor function in retinoblastoma cells. Investigative Ophthalmology and Visual Science. 2009;**50**:4542-4551

[59] Jo DH, Kim JH, Park WY, Kim KW, Yu YS. Differential profiles of microRNAs in retinoblastoma cell lines of different proliferation and adherence patterns. Journal of Pediatric Hematology/Oncology. 2011;**33**:529-533

[60] Asnaghi L, White DT, Key N, Choi J, Mahale A, Alkatan H, et al. ACVR1C/SMAD2 signaling promotes invasion and growth in retinoblastoma. Oncogene. 2019;**38**(12):2056-2075

[61] Greger V, Passarge E, Höpping W, Messmer E, Horsthemke B. Epigenetic changes may contribute to the formation and spontaneous regression of retinoblastoma. Human Genetics. 1989;**83**:155-158

[62] Ohtani-Fujita N, Dryja TP, Rapaport JM, Fujita T, Matsumura S, et al. Hypermethylation in the retinoblastoma gene is associated with unilateral, sporadic retinoblastoma. Cancer Genetics and Cytogenetics. 1997;**98**:43-49

[63] Richter S, Vandezande K, Chen N, Zhang K, Sutherland J, et al. Sensitive and efficient detection of *RB1 gene* mutations enhances care for families with retinoblastoma. American Journal of Human Genetics. 2003;**72**:253-269

[64] Livide G, Epistolato MC, Amenduni M, Disciglio V, Marozza A, et al. Epigenetic and copy number variation analysis in retinoblastoma by MS-MLPA. Pathology Oncology Research. 2012;**18**:703-712

[65] Harada K, Toyooka S, Maitra A, Maruyama R, Toyooka KO, et al. Aberrantpromotermethylation and silencing of the RASSF1A gene in pediatric tumors and cell lines. Oncogene. 2002;**21**:4345-4349

[66] Choy KW, Lee TC, Cheung KF, Fan DS, Lo KW, et al. Clinical implications of promoter hypermethylation in RASSF1A and MGMT in retinoblastoma. Neoplasia. 2005;**7**:200-206

[67] Bojinova RI, Schorderet DF, Addor MC, et al. Further delineation of the facial 13q14 deletion syndrome in 13 retinoblastoma patients. Ophthalmic Genetics. 2001;**22**:11-18

[68] Baud O, Cormier-Daire V, Lyonnet S, et al. Dysmorphic phenotype and neurological impairment in 22 retinoblastoma patients with constitutional cytogenetic 13q deletion. Clinical Genetics. 1999;**55**:478-482

[69] Jurkiewicz E, Pakula-Kosciesza I, Rutynowska O, et al. Trilateral retinoblastoma: An institutional experience and review of the literature. Child's Nervous System. 2010;**26**:129-132

[70] Kivela T. Trilateral retinoblastoma: A meta-analysis of hereditary

retinoblastoma associated with primary ectopic intracranial retinoblastoma. Journal of Clinical Oncology. 1999;**17**:1829-1837

[71] Singh AD, Shields CL, Shields JA. New insights into trilateral retinoblastoma. Cancer. 1999;**86**:3-5

[72] Kleinerman RA, Yu CL, Little MP, et al. Variation of second cancer risk by family history of retinoblastoma among long-term survivors. Journal of Clinical Oncology. 2012;**30**:950-957

[73] Ahmad NN, Melo MB, Singh AD, Donoso LA, Shields JA. A possible hot spot in exon 21 of the retinoblastoma gene predisposing to a low penetrant retinoblastoma phenotype? Ophthalmic Genetics. 1999;**20**:225-231

[74] Mallipatna A, Gallie BL, Chévez-Barrios P, Lumbroso-Le Rouic L, Chantada GL, Doz F, et al. Retinoblastoma. In: Amin MB, Edge SB, Greene FL, editors. AJCC Cancer Staging Manual. 8th ed. New York, NY: Springer; 2017. pp. 819-831

[75] Soliman SE, Racher H, Zhang C, MacDonald H, Gallie BL. Genetics and molecular diagnostics in retinoblastoma--an update. Asia-Pacific Journal of Ophthalmology. 2017a;**6**:197-207

[76] Sippel KC, Fraioli RE, Smith GD, Schalkoff ME, Sutherland J, Gallie BL, et al. Frequency of somatic and germ-line mosaicism in retinoblastoma: Implications for genetic counseling. American Journal of Human Genetics. 1998;**62**(3):610-619

[77] Rushlow DE, Mol BM, Kennett JY, Yee S, Pajovic S, Thériault BL, et al. Characterisation of retinoblastomas without RB1 mutations: Genomic, gene expression, and clinical studies. The Lancet Oncology. 2013;**14**:327-334

[78] Batzir NA, Shohat M, Maya I. Chromosomal microarray analysis (CMA) a clinical diagnostic tool in the prenatal and postnatal settings. Pediatric Endocrinology Reviews. 2015 Sep;**13**(1):448-454

[79] Mitter D, Ullmann R, Muradyan A, Klein-Hitpass L, Kanber D, Ounap K, et al. Genotype-phenotype correlations in patients with retinoblastoma and interstitial 13q deletions. European Journal of Human Genetics. 2011;**19**:947-958

[80] Castéra L, Dehainault C, Michaux D, Lumbroso-Le Rouic L, Aerts I, Doz F, et al. Fine mapping of whole *RB1 gene* deletions in retinoblastoma patients confirms PCDH8 as a candidate gene for psychomotor delay. European Journal of Human Genetics. 2013;**21**:460-464

[81] Dhar SU, Chintagumpala M, Noll C, Chévez-Barrios P, Paysse EA, Plon SE. Outcomes of integrating genetics in management of patients with retinoblastoma. Archives of Ophthalmology. 2011;**129**(11):1428-1434

[82] Canadian Retinoblastoma Society. National Retinoblastoma Strategy Canadian Guidelines for Care: Stratégie Thérapeutique du Rétinoblastome Guide Clinique Canadien [Internet]. 2009. Accessed: 2-20-19

[83] Soliman SE, Dimaras H, Khetan V, Gardiner JA, Chan HS, Héon E, et al. Prenatal versus postnatal screening for familial retinoblastoma. Ophthalmology. 2016;**123**:2610-2617

[84] Paquette LB, Miller D, Jackson HA, Lee T, Randolph L, Murphree AL, et al. In utero detection of retinoblastoma with fetal magnetic resonance and ultrasound: Initial experience. AJP Reports. 2012;**2**(1):55-62. DOI: 10.1055/s-0032-1316465

[85] Soliman S, Kletke S, Roelofs K, VandenHoven C, McKeen L, Gallie B. Precision laser therapy for

retinoblastoma. Expert Review of Ophthalmology. 2018;**13**:149-159

[86] Valenzuela AA, Chan HSL, Gallie BL. A language for retinoblastoma: Guidelines through standard operating procedures. In: Reynolds JD, editor. Pediatric Retina. New York: Spinger; 2011. pp. 205-234

[87] Temming P, Arendt M, Viehmann A, et al. How eye-preserving therapy affects long-term overall survival in heritable retinoblastoma survivors. Journal of Clinical Oncology. 2016;**34**:3183-3188

[88] Abramson DH, Mendelsohn ME, Servodidio CA, Tretter T, Gombos DS. Familial retinoblastoma: Where and when? Acta Ophthalmologica Scandinavica. 1998;**76**(3):334-338

Chapter 2

Epidemiological and Genetic Considerations in Retinoblastoma

Ido Didi Fabian, Faisal Al Qahtani and Covadonga Bascaran

Abstract

Retinoblastoma (Rb) is the most common primary intraocular malignancy of childhood. The incidence of Rb is stable worldwide at one case per 16,000–18,000 live births. It is estimated that 7800–8800 Rb cases were newly diagnosed globally in 2017. Over 80% of these are in low- and middle-income countries (LMICs) in Asia and Africa. So far, there is no validated evidence that retinoblastoma incidence is associated with gender, ethnicity or geographical factors. A link between human papillomavirus (HPV) and Rb is being investigated to establish its role in the pathophysiology of the sporadic form of the disease. Survival rates for Rb vary greatly between countries: while almost all Rb cases from high-income countries survive, cases in LMICs have a mortality rate of up to 70%.

Keywords: retinoblastoma, incidence, *RB1*, hereditary

1. Introduction

Retinoblastoma (Rb) is the most common intraocular malignancy of childhood, but a relatively rare disease, occurring in approximately 1: 16,000–18,000 live births [1]. Its incidence is uniform across populations, with no known gender, racial or ethnic predilection. Rb develops in early childhood, with the vast majority of cases that present before the age of 5 years. The disease can involve one or both eyes and can be inherited from an affected parent or developed *de novo* in a child with no family history of Rb. This chapter discusses the epidemiological aspects of Rb, including basic concepts in Rb development, incidence and prevalence, age, sex and racial considerations, associated environmental factors, trilateral Rb and secondary non-Rb malignancies.

2. Genetic considerations

Rb can be inherited by an affected parent or developed *de novo* in a child with no known family history of Rb (i.e., sporadic). The neoplasm can involve one or both eyes and may present in an asymmetrical manner, with different grades in each eye at presentation or even initially appearing as unilateral and becoming bilateral in the course of the disease. The disorder, which is believed to originate from an immature cone photoreceptor cell early in childhood, is initiated in most cases by a mutation in the *RB1* gene. *RB1* loss initially produces a retinoma, the benign precursor of Rb, and causes genomic instability that subsequently leads to the cancerous tumor, Rb.

In hereditary Rb cases, a single *RB1* allele is mutated in most or every cell of a child's body. An additional "hit" in the second allele in the retina will result in clinical Rb. These cases usually present with bilateral and multifocal disease at a median age of 15 months, but can present also in unilateral disease, albeit less frequently. Between 30 and 37% of Rb cases are bilateral [2], and all bilateral cases are hereditary. However, it is estimated that up to 18% of unilateral cases are also hereditary [3]. This emphasizes the importance of genetic testing in addition to clinical examination, as it has direct impact on the recommended screening frequency of the fellow eye and occasionally on management decisions.

Non-hereditary cases (i.e., somatic) usually present at a later age (median: 24 months) with unilateral unifocal disease. In order for the disease to develop in this scenario, two consecutive "hits" occur in a retinal cell, resulting in both *RB1* alleles mutated and the development of clinical Rb.

All familial cases are hereditary, but not necessarily vice versa. A mutation can occur at or after conception in an individual with no family history of Rb, and depending on the stage at which it occurs, some of the fetus' cells will have a mutated *RB1* allele, resulting in mosaicism. Children with mosaicism are at increased risk of developing Rb. The disease in this scenario is not inherited, hence siblings of the proband are not at risk, but offspring potentially are, and therefore should be screened soon after birth.

Hereditary Rb has been associated with an increased risk of developing secondary non-Rb malignancies [4, 5], including sarcomas, carcinomas, malignant melanoma, and neuroectodermal cancers. Secondary tumors were reported to occur in up to 20% of cases in 10 years and the incidence was reported to directly correlate with the time lag from initial diagnosis. It is also well established that treatment by radiotherapy increases the risk of developing secondary tumors, both in and outside the field of radiation [6]. Draper et al. showed in a series of nearly 400 hereditary cases that close to 10% developed secondary malignancies, mainly osteosarcomas, most of which were in the field of radiation [6].

Trilateral Rb is a syndrome consisting of unilateral or bilateral hereditary Rb associated with an intracranial neuroblastic tumor that develops most often in the pineal gland (i.e., Pinealblastoma). On a meta-analysis by Kivelä [7], 2% of trilateral Rb cases had a brain tumor but no intraocular Rb, 12% had unilateral Rb and the remaining had bilateral disease.

3. Magnitude and distribution of Rb

3.1 Global incidence and prevalence

The reported incidence of Rb is constant worldwide at one case per 16,000–18,000 live births [8, 9]. In 2009 the estimated global annual incidence of Rb ranged from 7200 to 8100 children. The global birth rate has dropped since then, from 20.3 to 18.6 births per 1000 population, but the world's population has grown from 6593 to 7550 million [10], resulting in an estimated 7800–8800 newly diagnosed Rb cases globally in 2017. The highest disease prevalence is recorded in areas with high birth rates, which is the case of many low- and middle-income countries (LMICs).

3.2 Global distribution and survival

Over 80% of the newly diagnosed cases are in LMICs in Asia and Africa (**Table 1** and **Figure 1**) [3]. These regions also show the lowest survival rate, reporting up to 70% mortality from Rb. Only about 15% of children with Rb reside in high-income

	High incidence (1:16,000)	Low incidence (1:18,000)	Average incidence
	n	*n*	*n* (%)
Continent			
North America	273	242	258 (3.1)
Latin America and the Caribbean	669	595	632 (7.7)
Africa	2567	2282	2425 (29.5)
Asia	4656	4139	4398 (53.5)
Europe	504	448	476 (5.8)
Oceania	37	32	35 (0.4)
National income level			
Low	1413	1256	1335 (16.2)
Lower-middle	4221	3752	3987 (48.5)
Upper-middle	2272	2020	2146 (26.1)
High	800	711	756 (9.2)

Table 1.
Estimated number of newly diagnosed retinoblastoma patients in 2017.

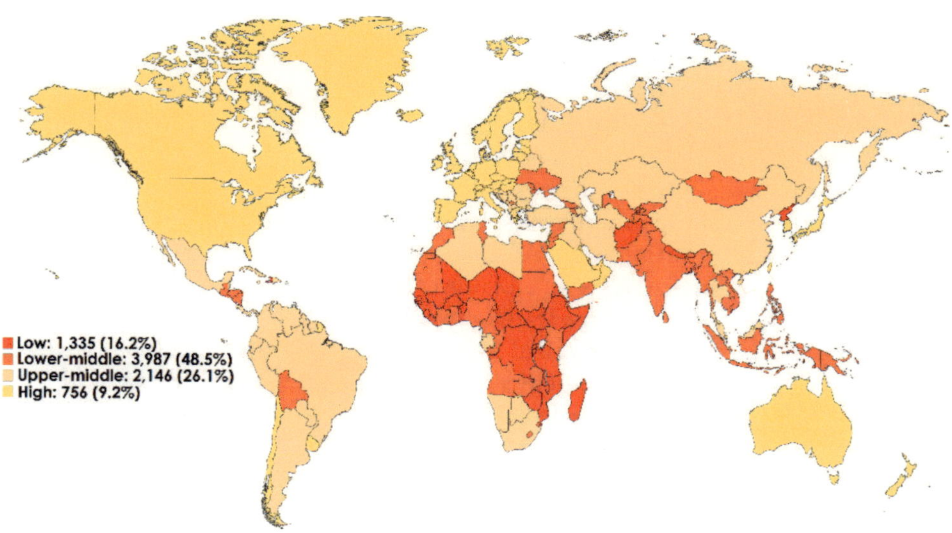

Figure 1.
Estimated average number of newly diagnosed Rb patients in 2017 by national income level. Income level data source: United Nations, Department of Economic and Social Affairs PD [10].

countries, and their prognosis is considered to be very good, with an estimated disease-free survival rate of nearly 100% [11].

4. Rb determinants

4.1 Age

According to the World Health Organization's compendium of data from cancer registries, the average Rb incidence rate in children aged 0–4 years is >10 per million compared to <1 per million in children aged 5–9 years, and significantly lower beyond that age [12].

It is difficult to accurately estimate the time at which Rb tumors first develop as information about the biological development of the disease is essentially lacking. There are three important time points associated with Rb development and the time of Rb diagnosis. These include (1) retinal tumor growth following two *RB1* mutative events, (2) parents/guardians noticing the first ocular sign, and (3) presentation to an Rb center, at which diagnosis is made and treatment given.

As discussed earlier, the median age of presentation for bilateral cases is 15 months, while for non-hereditary cases is 24 months. Most of the available knowledge originates from familial cases in high income countries, where Rb centers commonly perform screening tests for patients at risk (i.e., siblings of probands). Screening allows detection of small tumors very early in the course of disease, relatively soon after they develop. However, since sporadic cases are not screened, we rely only on age of presentation at two time points. First, the time at which the parents/guardians notice an ocular abnormality, it is usually a white pupillary reflex (i.e., leukocoria). Second, the time at which the final diagnosis is made, which is dependent on the time it takes the patient to reach the Rb center in the referral pathway.

The body of knowledge on Rb is based on retrospective studies, hence, the most accurate data in this context reports the age of the child's first presentation at an Rb center. Nevertheless, several studies have investigated the lag time from the first ocular sign as noticed by parents, to the presenting sign at the Rb center. In this respect, a huge gap exists between high-income countries and LMICs. In the UK, the referral time from sign onset to visiting primary care was found to be 28 days, primary care to ophthalmologist 3 days, and the time from local ophthalmologist to an Rb Unit was 6 days. In low-income countries, these time lags are considerably longer, and can take 6 months or more [13].

Rarely, Rb can develop in adults older than 20 years of age, with fewer than 50 case reports found in the literature. Adult-onset Rb is quite different in its presentation compared to its pediatric form, and due to its rarity, it is usually not considered in the differential diagnosis, often leading to delay in diagnosis.

In trilateral Rb [7], rates of familial Rb, the age at diagnosis and laterality were found to be similar to ordinary hereditary Rb. Cases of suprasellar trilateral Rb, however, were diagnosed at an earlier age as compared to Pinealblastoma. The median age of Rb diagnosis was 5 months, and cases of familial Rb were diagnosed at an earlier age than non-familial cases.

4.2 Gender

There is no known gender predilection in Rb, and although this notion is widely quoted in many scientific reports in the field, it has not actually been thoroughly investigated. Based on data available from the Surveillance, Epidemiology, and End Results (SEER) program of the National Cancer Institute, Tamboli et al. calculated the incidence of Rb in the United States from 1974 to 1985 and found no gender differences [14]. Gurney et al. used the same data source for similar years (1974–1989), but concluded that rates of Rb were higher in females [15], and Wong et al., in contrast, found an excess of Rb cases in males using the SEER database for the years 2000–2009 [8]. *RB1* gene is located on chromosome 13 and there is no known relation to any of the sex chromosomes. There is also no evidence of an association between sex hormones and Rb. Cases of trilateral Rb do not show any gender predilection either [7].

4.3 Race

Similar to sex, there is no known association between race and Rb, although some exceptions have been reported. Gurney et al. found higher rates of Rb in blacks as compared to whites in the United States [15]. Broaddus et al., in contrast, found that the overall mean age-adjusted incidence of Rb was 11.3 for Caucasians and 13.0 for blacks, with no significant difference between the two populations [8]. Krishna et al. examined the incidence of Rb using data from the International Agency for Research on Cancer [16], and found no significant difference between white populations in the United States and Europe/Australia, Hispanic populations in Spain and the United States, and Hispanic populations in Uruguay and the United States. They concluded that Rb incidence is similar among varied populations.

4.4 Environmental factors

Several studies have shown a link between human papillomavirus (HPV) and the development of sporadic Rb [17, 18]. Shetty et al. analyzed enucleated eyes with Rb and found that 70% were positive for HPV [17], suggesting that the virus may play a role in the development of sporadic RB. Anand et al. tested the presence of HPV in Rb tissue (formalin-fixed paraffin-embedded tissue and fresh-frozen specimens) and found that nearly a quarter of the specimens were positive for HPV [19]. However, the implications of the presence of HPV in Rb tissue and its role in carcinogenesis warrant further study. Jemal et al. investigated the relation between Rb incidence and ultraviolet (UV-B) radiation levels in the SEER program and found no statistically significant correlations [20]. To the best of our knowledge, there are no other reports focused on any additional environmental factors in association with Rb development.

5. Conclusions

Rb is the most common primary intraocular malignancy of childhood. The disease can involve one or both eyes and can be inherited or sporadic. The incidence of Rb is stable worldwide at one case per 16,000–18,000 live births. The average Rb incidence rate in children aged 0–4 years is >10 per million compared to <1 per million in children aged 5–9 years, and significantly lower beyond that age. In 2017, globally, an estimated 7800–8800 Rb cases were newly diagnosed. Over 80% of these are in LMICs in Asia and Africa.

So far, there is no validated evidence that retinoblastoma incidence is associated with gender, ethnicity or geographical factors. Studies have shown the presence of HPV in sporadic Rb tissue. Its role in carcinogenesis and the development of sporadic Rb warrants further investigation.

We lack accurate information about the biological development of Rb which creates difficulties in estimating the time at which Rb tumors first develop. In familial cases from high-income countries, genetic screening is routinely conducted. However, in low-income countries this is not the case, and in all settings sporadic cases are not screened. In these cases, we rely on time of presentation, which is strongly influenced by the referral pathways in different settings.

Survival rates are related to the time taken for the child to present at an Rb center and vary greatly between countries: while almost all Rb cases from high-income countries survive, cases in LMICs have a mortality rate of 70%.

Conflict of interest

No conflicts of interest to disclose.

Author details

Ido Didi Fabian[1*], Faisal Al Qahtani[2] and Covadonga Bascaran[1]

1 International Centre for Eye Health, London School of Hygiene and Tropical Medicine, London, UK

2 King Saud University, Riyadh, Saudi Arabia

*Address all correspondence to: didi@didifabian.com

References

[1] Kivelä T. The epidemiological challenge of the most frequent eye cancer: Retinoblastoma, an issue of birth and death. The British Journal of Ophthalmology. 2009;**93**:1129-1131. DOI: 10.1136/bjo.2008.150292

[2] MacCarthy A, Birch JM, Draper GJ, et al. Retinoblastoma in Great Britain 1963-2002. The British Journal of Ophthalmology. 2009;**93**:33-37. DOI: 10.1136/bjo.2008.139618

[3] Dimaras H, Corson TW, Cobrinik D, et al. Retinoblastoma. Nature Reviews. Disease Primers. 2015;**1**:15021. DOI: 10.1038/nrdp.2015.21

[4] Smith LM, Donaldson SS, Egbert PR, et al. Aggressive management of second primary tumors in survivors of hereditary retinoblastoma. International Journal of Radiation Oncology, Biology, Physics. 1989;**17**:499-505. Available from: http://www.ncbi.nlm.nih.gov/pubmed/2777644 [Accessed: 27 February 2019]

[5] Abramson DH, Ellsworth RM, Kitchin FD, et al. Second nonocular tumors in retinoblastoma survivors. Are they radiation-induced? Ophthalmology. 1984;**91**:1351-1355. Available from: http://www.ncbi.nlm.nih.gov/pubmed/6595610 [Accessed: 27 February 2019]

[6] Draper GJ, Sanders BM, Kingston JE. Second primary neoplasms in patients with retinoblastoma. British Journal of Cancer. 1986;**53**:661-671. Available from: http://www.ncbi.nlm.nih.gov/pubmed/3718823 [Accessed: 27 February 2019]

[7] Kivelä T. Trilateral retinoblastoma: A meta-analysis of hereditary retinoblastoma associated with primary ectopic intracranial retinoblastoma. Journal of Clinical Oncology. 1999;**17**:1829-1837. DOI: 10.1200/JCO.1999.17.6.1829

[8] Broaddus E, Topham A, Singh AD. Incidence of retinoblastoma in the USA: 1975-2004. The British Journal of Ophthalmology. 2009;**93**:21-23. DOI: 10.1136/bjo.2008.138750

[9] Seregard S, Lundell G, Svedberg H, et al. Incidence of retinoblastoma from 1958 to 1998 in Northern Europe. Advantages of birth cohort analysis. Ophthalmology. 2004;**111**:1228-1232. DOI: 10.1016/j.ophtha.2003.10.023

[10] United Nations, Department of Economic and Social Affairs Population Division. World Population Prospects the 2017 Revision. Vol. I: Comprehensive Tables (ST/ESA/SER.A/399). 2017. Available from: https://esa.un.org/unpd/wpp/Publications/Files/WPP2017_Volume-I_Comprehensive-Tables.pdf [Accessed: 29 November 2017]

[11] MacCarthy A, Birch JM, Draper GJ, et al. Retinoblastoma: Treatment and survival in Great Britain 1963 to 2002. The British Journal of Ophthalmology. 2009;**93**:38-39. DOI: 10.1136/bjo.2008.139626

[12] International Agency for Research on Cancer. International Incidence of Childhood Cancer International Agency for Research on Cancer. Lyon, France. 1998. Available from: http://iicc.iarc.fr/results/

[13] Sitorus RS, Moll AC, Suhardjono S, et al. The effect of therapy refusal against medical advice in retinoblastoma patients in a setting where treatment delays are common. Ophthalmic Genetics. 2009;**30**:31-36. DOI: 10.1080/13816810802464320

[14] Tamboli A, Podgor MJ, Horm JW. The incidence of retinoblastoma in the United States: 1974 through 1985. Archives of Ophthalmology (Chicago, Ill: 1960). 1990;**108**:128-132. Available from: http://www.ncbi.nlm.nih.

gov/pubmed/2288550 [Accessed: 13 February 2019]

[15] Gurney JG, Severson RK, Davis S, et al. Incidence of cancer in children in the United States. Sex-, race-, and 1-year age-specific rates by histologic type. Cancer. 1995;**75**:2186-2195. Available from: http://www.ncbi.nlm.nih.gov/pubmed/7697611 [Accessed: 13 February 2019]

[16] Krishna SM, Yu G-P, Finger PT. The effect of race on the incidence of retinoblastoma. Journal of Pediatric Ophthalmology and Strabismus. 2009;**46**:288-293. DOI: 10.3928/01913913-20090903-06

[17] Shetty OA, Naresh KN, Banavali SD, et al. Evidence for the presence of high risk human papillomavirus in retinoblastoma tissue from nonfamilial retinoblastoma in developing countries. Pediatric Blood & Cancer. 2012;**58**:185-190. DOI: 10.1002/pbc.23346

[18] Orjuela M, Castaneda VP, Ridaura C, et al. Presence of human papilloma virus in tumor tissue from children with retinoblastoma: An alternative mechanism for tumor development. Clinical Cancer Research. 2000;**6**:4010-4016. Available from: http://www.ncbi.nlm.nih.gov/pubmed/11051250 [Accessed: 25 February 2019]

[19] Anand B, Ramesh C, Appaji L, et al. Prevalence of high-risk human papillomavirus genotypes in retinoblastoma. The British Journal of Ophthalmology. 2011;**95**:1014-1018. DOI: 10.1136/bjo.2010.199802

[20] Jemal A, Devesa SS, Fears TR, et al. Retinoblastoma incidence and sunlight exposure. British Journal of Cancer. 2000;**82**:1875-1878. DOI: 10.1054/bjoc.2000.1215

Section 2

Clinical Aspects, Management and Prognosis

Chapter 3

Retinoblastoma: Presentation, Evaluation, and Diagnosis

Spencer T. Langevin and Brian P. Marr

Abstract

Retinoblastoma was initially described in a case series by Dr. James Wardrop in 1809. Since then, the evaluation and diagnosis of retinoblastoma has progressed significantly, thus providing a framework for successful therapy with up to 97% survival rate in developed nations. Here we outline the presentation, evaluation, and detailed diagnostic steps of any child presenting with signs and symptoms of retinoblastoma (RB). We detail the questions and pertinent history to obtain, describe in detail the examination under anesthesia, ancillary testing, and recommendations for both anesthesia and neuroimaging. We also cover the differential diagnosis of retinoblastoma and the most common simulating lesions to present to an ophthalmologist. We describe the ways to determine if a patient has retinoblastoma or some simulating lesion, and the characteristics associated with each possibility. Finally, we briefly address genetic counseling and the next steps after diagnosis.

Keywords: retinoblastoma, intraocular tumors, oncology, children, b-scan ultrasonography, leukocoria, evaluation, diagnosis

1. Introduction

Pawius of Amsterdam is the first physician credited with recognizing retinoblastoma in the autopsy of a young child in 1597 [1]. In 1809, a Scottish surgeon from Edinburgh, James Wardrop, published a monograph entitled "*Observations on the fungus haematodes, or soft cancer, in several of the most important organs of the human body*". His monograph included clinical histories of 15 children diagnosed with an intraocular tumor at the age of 1–6 years [2]. Dr. Wardrop described the tumors as "white in colour and brain-like in substance", and he concluded as well that they were of retinal origin. He even went so far as to recommend enucleation to save the life of the children, in which his peers did not agree with him at the time. The first case in American literature was by Dr. Steven at New York Hospital in 1818 [3]. At the time, retinoblastoma was known at *fungus haematodes* which was initially described by Dr. Hey of Leeds, England [4]. Virchow in 1845 renamed the entity *glioma of the retina* [5]. Hirschberg further described the glioma into *exophytum* and *endophytum* [6]. Flexner described the histologic findings of cellular rosettes in the tumor in 1891 [7]. In 1897, Wintersteiner described the lumen of the rosette [8]. Finally Verhoeff named the tumor *retinoblastoma* which was adopted by the American Ophthalmological Society in 1926, thus arriving at the terminology we use to this day [9].

2. Presentation, evaluation, and diagnosis

2.1 Clinical presentation

The initial signs and symptoms of retinoblastoma (RB) are usually noticed by friends or family members, or at times from an abnormal "red reflex", more specifically, a white reflex or (leukocoria) from a photograph. Medical professionals, such as pediatricians during a routine examination, or a pediatric ophthalmologist, may also notice signs and symptoms consistent with RB, however less often. In very rare circumstances the intraocular mass may be picked up on head imaging for non-ophthalmic reasons. In developed nations such as the United States, the most common presenting finding for intraocular retinoblastoma is leukocoria or "cats eye reflex" (43%), followed by strabismus (22%), pseudo cellulitis, (9%), microphthalmia (5%), routine screening examination (17%), and rarely the presence of an intraocular mass on non-ophthalmic imaging (<1%) [10].

On average the ophthalmic oncologist is the third medical professional to evaluate a child suspicious for having RB. According to a large study on referral patterns there is an average delay of 1.1 months between initial symptoms and evaluation with any medical professional, and 2.0 months before an appointment with an ophthalmic oncologist [10]. As of 2014, mortality from retinoblastoma in the United States is approximately 3%, however in developing countries is close to 60%. Although our treatment has improved greatly, in many parts of the world access to care is a large barrier to successful therapy. Mean age at diagnosis in Asia is 22 months, compared to North America and Europe which are 12 and 9 months, respectively. On a more significant note, there are approximately 3000 new cases of retinoblastoma in Asia compared to only 300 new cases in North America, even further highlighting the need for improved access to care. As there are relatively few specialists and centers who treat such a rare condition, it is important to use the internet, telemedicine, and other social services to help train ancillary staff and improve access to triage services to improve prognosis for children.

2.2 Misdiagnosis and differential diagnosis

A review of the literature demonstrates a historic misdiagnosis rate of 11–40% based on histopathologic analysis of enucleated specimens, and a clinical misdiagnosis rate from 16 to 53% [10]. Fortunately the accuracy in diagnosis at specialized ophthalmic oncology centers in the United States is believed to exceed 99%. In a recent review of referring physician patterns the most common simulating lesions (>5% of analyzed lesions) were: Persistent fetal vasculature, Coat's Disease, Astrocytic Hamartoma, Intraretinal hemorrhage, and retinal detachment. Retinopathy of prematurity and congenital cataract were previously misdiagnosed often, but increased awareness of these conditions and better examination practices are likely the cause of reduced misdiagnosis of these two entities. Misdiagnosis of RB may be due to the fact that the condition is exceedingly rare, large differential diagnosis, and the challenges of examining children. Thus, any suspicion for the condition should warrant prompt referral to specialized care [11].

2.3 Evaluation and diagnosis of retinoblastoma

We will describe an organized approach in a stepwise manner for evaluating and properly diagnosis of RB. This will consist of: detailed history, initial office examination, ultrasonographic testing, examination under anesthesia, and current consensus on imaging and genetic testing. Modifications dependent on specific patient encounters should be left to the treating physician.

2.3.1 History

For any child with suspicion of retinoblastoma, a very detailed history is the most useful step in establishing an appropriate differential diagnosis and accurate examination, and in cases may establish the diagnosis. History should be taken prior to examination to ensure an appropriate focused examination. It should include details of the pregnancy, labor, and delivery of the child. History of birth weight, birth trauma, maternal infection, history of prematurity, oxygen therapy, and whether leukocoria was present at birth or developed later. Also, history of hearing abnormalities at birth or during young childhood should be taken into consideration as well. History of animal/pet exposure should also be elicited. These questions should help direct the clinician to the diagnosis of cataract, retinopathy of prematurity, persistent fetal vasculature, toxocariasis, and congenital rubella, which all can mimic retinoblastoma. The time course of when parents or clinicians first noticed an abnormality and the course of their visits with other health care providers should be carefully elicited. Most children with retinoblastoma do not have an obvious ocular abnormality at birth. They tend to develop signs such as esotropia, visual disturbances, or other strabismus between 6 months and 2 years of age. Leukocoria is also unlikely to be present at birth and will occur around the same time frame as the strabismus. For children suspected to have retinoblastoma a detailed family history including number and health of their siblings should be noted, along with any history of family medical conditions. A history of poor vision, blindness, or loss of an eye should be requested. A positive history of retinoblastoma in parents should point to the diagnosis, as simulating lesions do not usually occur in patients with a positive family history. If the child's parents or siblings have not had recent dilated fundus examinations they should be performed as soon as possible [12]. About 1% of patients with history of retinoblastoma may develop spontaneous regression with retinoma/ retinocytoma present on dilated examination [13]. Some parents may be unaware that they were treated for retinoblastoma as children and examination may be able to elicit this finding.

2.3.2 Office examination

The initial examination of the child should occur while history taking, by watching the child's behavior, visual interaction with the world, and evaluating for any abnormalities in size of the child, proportions, or for any facial abnormalities. The external examination of a child with retinoblastoma should be otherwise normal except for the ocular exam unless the child has a 13q deletion syndrome. Before the formal examination, the ability to notice leukocoria, decreased visual function, strabismus, or periorbital swelling should be noted upon gross examination. Assessment of vision is obviously dependent on age of patient, and his or her individual cooperation, but the size and symmetry of each eye should be recorded, as asymmetric size can suggest other diagnoses as well as retinoblastoma. Presence or absence of heterochromia should be noted during this portion of the examination as well [12]. Pupil response should also be documented. Using a direct ophthalmoscope or retinoscope, the pupillary light reflex should be noted in both eyes and leukocoria can be noted at that time.

The next step should be instillation of dilating eyedrops (0.5% tropicamide and 2.5% phenylephrine). Cyclopentolate is not necessary for this examination. If the child is large enough or a portable slit lamp is available, slit lamp examination should be performed, care to note, presence or absence of cataract, conjunctival or scleral injection, anterior segment shallowing, neovascularization of the iris, iris seeding or iris atrophy. Evaluate for retrolental membranes to assess presence of retinopathy of prematurity or persistent fetal vasculature. Most patients with retinoblastoma have normal anterior segments but may have anterior cells or nodules on the iris. In exophytic tumors, visualization of retinal vasculature behind the lens may be possible as well. Indirect ophthalmoscopy should be performed to evaluate the posterior pole and fundus. Depending on the age of the child, they may cooperate or family members may be needed to help secure the patient in a supine position. Very young children may be swaddled with a blanket to secure their limbs. The indirect exam in the office should be used to rule out simulating lesions when possible and to also increase or decrease suspicion for retinoblastoma, thus determining whether examination under anesthesia (EUA) is needed for full evaluation and diagnosis. An eyelid speculum may be needed for proper dilated examination, and a topical anesthetic such as 0.5 or 1% proparacaine should be instilled prior to speculum insertion. Scleral depression may be indicated, if it can be reserved for examination under anesthesia it is less traumatic but can be done in the office setting.

2.3.3 Ophthalmic ultrasound

An ophthalmic ultrasound can be performed in the A and B scan mode using a 10 mHz transducer to evaluate for intraocular masses, retinal detachment, or calcification. In retinoblastoma, the ultrasound should reveal an irregular mass, which is more echogenic than the vitreous, and commonly has fine calcifications (highly reflective foci mostly with acoustic shadowing) since upon histologic study, 95% of retinoblastoma contains calcification [14] (**Figure 1**). Measurements should be taken as a baseline to compare to in the future following treatment.

2.4 Exam under anesthesia (EUA) considerations

If EUA is warranted, general anesthesia will be needed to conduct detailed examination and ancillary testing at one time. Preparation of the room for EUA should consist of examination materials including: external photography, portable slit lamp, tonometry, indirect ophthalmoscope with condensing lens and scleral

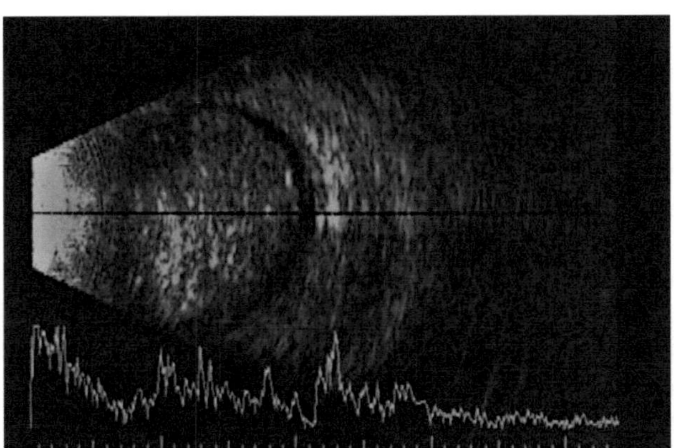

Figure 1.
10 mHz ultrasound in A and B scan mode showing a large intraocular retinoblastoma with irregular mass and intrinsic calcification with acoustic shadowing.

depressor, wide-angle hand-held fundus camera, intravenous fluorescein dye, high resolution ophthalmic ultrasound, ultrasound biomicroscopy, electroretinography. When retinoblastoma is confirmed, an MRI of the brain and orbits with and without contrast should be ordered at the time of the EUA to assess for extrascleral extension, orbital anatomy, posterior portion of the optic nerve, and presence of pinealoblastoma in trilateral disease.

2.5 Anesthesia

The type of general anesthetic and airway support varies depending on institution and available resources. Safe anesthesia methods range from mask anesthesia, to laryngeal mask airway (LMA), to complete endotracheal intubation. Both inhaled anesthetics and intravenous anesthetics, or a combination of the two, are suitable for examination. General guidelines recommend that heavy fatty meals be discontinued 8 h prior to procedure, light meals, formula, and nonhuman milk 6 h prior to surgery, human milk 4 h prior to anesthesia, and clear liquids 2 h prior to anesthesia [15]. These recommendations will vary by location and anesthesiologist, and type of anesthesia administered. Recently there has been literature support for use of LMA without placement of intravenous lines, which reduces total time under anesthesia without increased anesthesia complications, all of which were managed successfully without long term sequelae [16].

2.6 Examination under anesthesia

2.6.1 External examination

An orderly approach to the exam should be taken to efficiently access and treat the patient to avoid prolonged anesthesia exposure. The overall features of the child should be assessed, evaluating for any abnormalities that are consistent with retinoblastoma and a 13Q deletion syndrome which is strongly associated with retinoblastoma risk (**Figure 2**). Patient's with 13Q deletion syndrome may have hypotelorism, micrognathia, hypoplasia of midface, absent nasal bones, large ears, hypoplastic thumbs, cleft palate, or microcephaly [17].

2.6.2 Anterior examination

Intraocular pressures should be measured using Schiotz tonometer, tonopen, Perkins tonometer, or pneumotonometer. Elevated intraocular pressure in patients with retinoblastoma can be secondary to iris neovascularization or angle closure, and has been associated with increased risk of optic nerve invasion and metastatic disease [18].

After intraocular pressure is checked, corneal diameter should be measured with a caliper both in horizontal and vertical directions. Conditions such as persistent fetal vasculature (PFV) is associated with asymmetric corneal diameter size as well as eyes with congenitally elevated intraocular pressures can be associated with buphthalmos and increased corneal diameter.

A portable slit lamp should be used to assess the anterior segment. The clinician should evaluate anterior depth, clarity of the lens, neovascularization of the iris or atrophy, retrolental membrane, anterior chamber cells, nodules of the iris, or anterior vitreous seeds seen behind the lens. Presence of a pseudohypopyon should raise suspicion for endophytic tumor and anterior chamber seeing of cancer. It may be possible to visualize retinal vascular, retrolental masses, or retrolental membranes. Retrolental retinal tissue should reveal blood vessel branching patterns

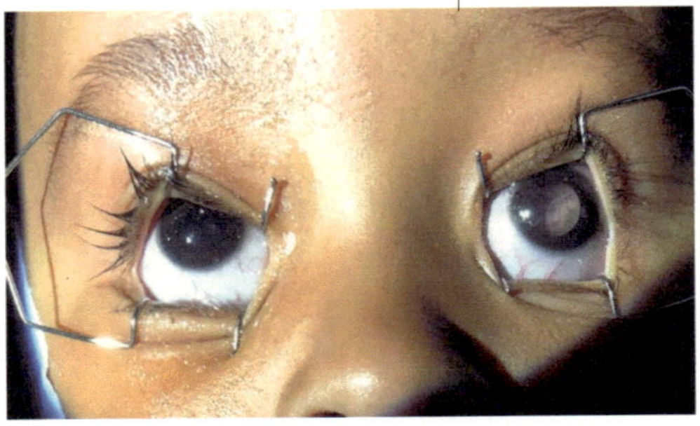

Figure 2.
External photograph of young child with leukocoria of the left eye secondary to intraocular retinoblastoma.

extending towards the periphery of the lens which could be secondary to exophytic tumor, whereas the persistent tunica vasculosa lentis in PFV, vessels should be noted to be growing towards the center of the posterior lens in a disorganized fashion. Retrolental membrane without vascular pattern is suggestive of retinopathy of prematurity rather than RB.

Binocular indirect ophthalmoscopy should then be performed in a step by step fashion. Initially the vitreous should be examined in both eyes for presence of seeding, vitreous hemorrhage, fibrous membranes, or inflammatory debris. If the posterior pole is visible, optic disc and macula should be examined and abnormal findings documented. Examination of the periphery should be performed with scleral depression of the ora serrata in a clockwise or counter-clockwise fashion, with examination of the midperipheral retina and posterior pole for 360 degrees in both eyes.

Small RB lesions can be difficult to detect as there can be poor contrast between the small translucent tumor and the surrounding fundus. Meticulous examination and depression is needed to observe these tumors stereoscopically. Medium sized tumors become more opaque and start appearing white. Large tumors (>4–5 mm) in diameter will begin to have visually obvious blood supply and visually significant feeder vessels should be noted. Many very large lesions (>6 mm) will develop chalky-white calcifications within the body of the tumor. The size and number of all tumors should be noted, with evaluation of subretinal fluid, retinal detachment, and presence of seeding (subretinal or vitreous) (**Figure 3**), and should all be incorporated into a detailed retinal drawing along with fundus photography [12]. Drawing and photography can help the clinician classify the tumor according to existing classification schemes at a later time.

2.6.3 Ancillary testing

2.6.3.1 Photography

It is important to obtain photographs of both the anterior segment as well as the vitreous cavity and posterior segment for documentation. The most useful method is using a wide-angle fundus camera. Photographs should be obtained during every EUA to help document response to therapy (**Figures 4**, **5A**, **B**, and **6A**, **B**). The clinician should try to standardize the photographs, so comparisons to each exam can be readily performed. As an example, start with a posterior pole photograph centered on the fovea then sequentially take peripheral photos superiorly, inferiorly, temporally and nasally keeping the optic nerve visible at the respective edge of the photograph to use as a point of reference for peripheral lesions. Then any other areas of special interest can be photographed separately.

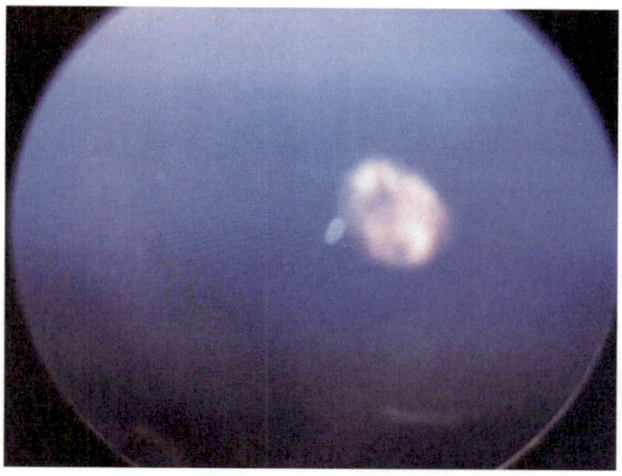

Figure 3.
RetCam photography of the left eye with defocusing to document free-floating vitreous seeding.

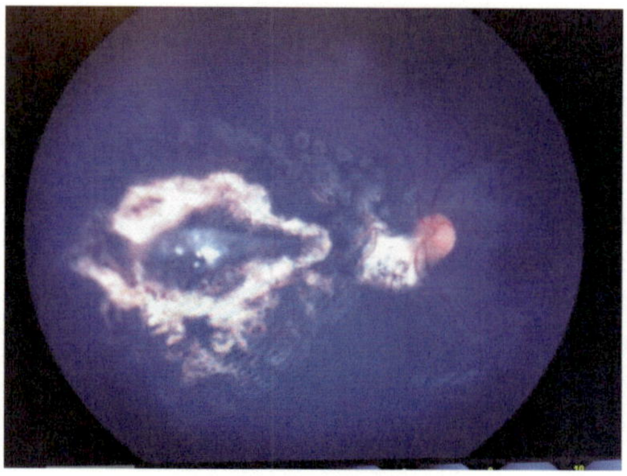

Figure 4.
A retinoblastoma of the left eye with tumor scar showing type 3 regression.

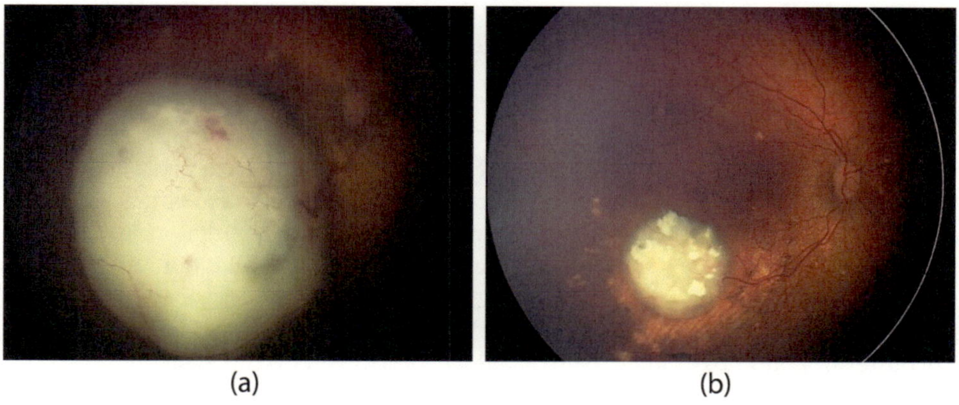

Figure 5.
(A) RetCam photograph of class C retinoblastoma of the right eye prior to intra-arterial chemotherapy and (B) RetCam photograph of the right eye showing class C retinoblastoma after treatment with intra-arterial chemotherapy.

2.6.3.2 Fluorescein angiography

Thanks to advances in photography as described in the above section, fluorescein angiography (FA) can be readily performed during an EUA and can help one

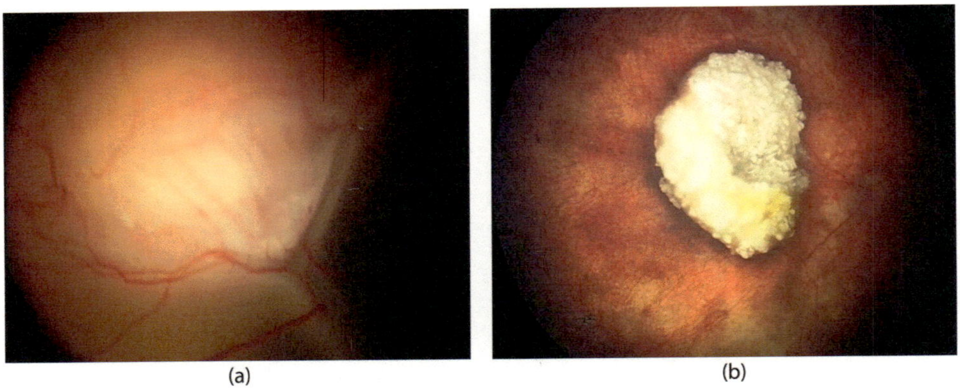

Figure 6.
(A) RetCam photograph of the left eye showing class D retinoblastoma prior to intra-arterial chemotherapy and (B) RetCam photograph of the left eye showing class D retinoblastoma after intra-arterial chemotherapy.

differentiate RB from simulating lesions. Firstly, subclinical neovascularization of the iris (NVI) can be distinguished using Retcam FA. In a recent study, eyes with advanced retinoblastoma, NVI was documented appearing as placoid or patchy areas of hyper fluorescence involving one or more sectors of the iris [19]. This finding typically occurred between 1 and 2 min. Retinoblastoma in the fundus should show dilated and tortuous vessels, with retinal arteries which "feed" the tumor of the largest caliber. Also, microaneurysms, retinal hemorrhages, and arteriovenous shunts can also be noted. In the same study, as the tumors enlarged, the abnormal vascularization was no longer consistent with normal retinal anatomy, and were contained entirely within the tumor itself. Intrinsic vessels of the tumor had disorganized and complex branching patterns, irregular caliber, and terminated early within the body of the tumor. This multi-level involvement of vascular abnormality helps the clinician readily distinguish RB from Coat's disease which has large dilated vessels which remain within one level of the retina and show extensive peripheral non-perfusion (**Figure 7A** and **B**). Lastly, after 3 min diffuse leakage from retinal vessels can lead to inability to discern fine details of the fundus, so the clinician should try to obtain all valuable information within the first 3 min of the study.

2.6.3.3 Ophthalmic ultrasonography

During the EUA, ultrasound imaging of both eyes can be used to assess the orbit for extraocular extension, to measure thickness of the lesions, and to obtain axial lengths of the eyes to evaluate for normal size and symmetry. Ophthalmic ultrasound has traditionally been used for diagnosing and monitoring treatment of retinoblastoma and distinguishing it from simulating lesions [20, 21]. As described previously in the chapter, a 10 mHz transducer in the A and B scan mode should be used to image the posterior pole and evaluate the size and location of tumors, evaluate for retinal detachment, and look for extraocular extension of tumor (**Figure 8**). Ultrasound is especially useful in cases when ophthalmoscopy is limited by a poor view or in presence of a cataract. As described previously in this chapter, large retinoblastoma lesions undergo dystrophic calcification from necrosis, and these can be readily observed as areas of hyper-reflection with acoustic shadowing.

2.6.3.4 Ultrasound biomicroscopy

Ultrasound biomicroscopy (UBM) can also be helpful for visualizing the iris, pars plana, pars plicata, and ciliary body during an EUA. It is extremely helpful to

DOI: http://dx.doi.org/10.5772/intechopen.85744

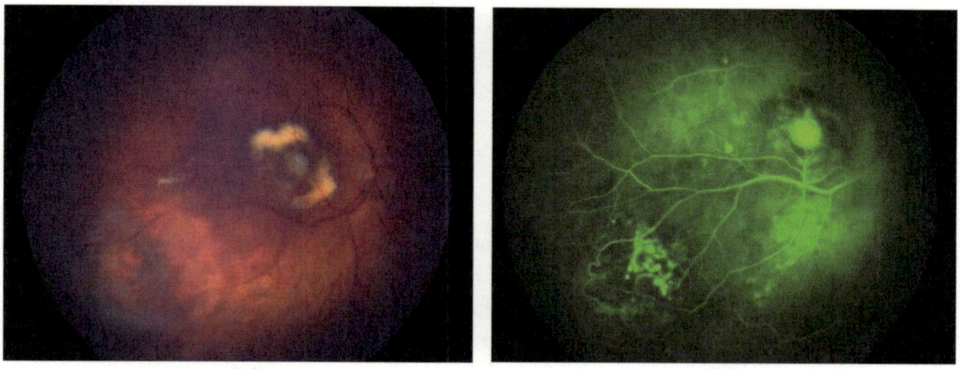

Figure 7.
(A) A portable wide field photograph showing a simulating lesion of retinoblastoma in the right eye showing a white macular lesion, close attention to the far periphery shows vascular telangiectasia and non-perfusion and (B) accompanying fluorescein angiogram confirming diagnosis of Coat's disease in 8 year old boy, again notice vascular telangiectasias and non-perfusion within a single plane of the retina.

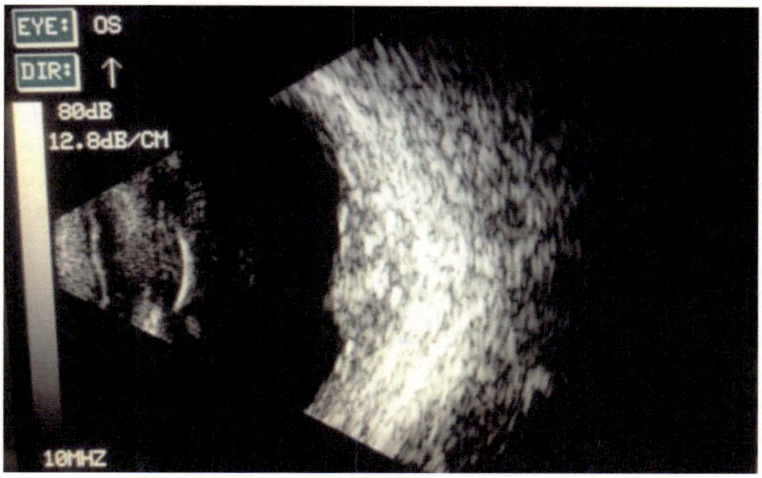

Figure 8.
10 mHz B-scan ultrasonography of the left eye showing treated intraocular retinoblastoma with intrinsic calcifications and acoustic shadowing.

assess the anterior extent of tumor burden or to obtain more information regarding the pars panna and ciliary body as well as anterior chamber seeding. It is especially important to use UBM to rule out pars plana tumor involvement in cases where intravitreal injections of chemotherapy are being considered to choose a proper injection site.

2.6.3.5 Electroretinogram

Electroretinograms (ERG) has been used to monitor retinal function before, during, and after therapy with intra-arterial chemotherapy. It is especially helpful in preverbal children who are unable to describe their level of visual function during the treatment course. Also it provides information regarding the cumulative effects of retinal damage secondary to therapy, chemotherapy toxicity, and tissue destruction from treatments including radiation, laser photocoagulation, and cryotherapy. During the EUA, a 30-Hz flicker has been tested and shown to be informative prior to the physical examination portion of the exam [22]. One must be cautious to not manipulate the eyes before obtaining the ERG, as ocular manipulation including scleral depression, photography, and ophthalmoscopy can affect the ERG readings thus confounding results [23].

2.6.3.6 Imaging for retinoblastoma

Historically computerized tomography (CT) scans were used to evaluate patients ocular, orbital, optic nerve, and brain involvement from the tumor, since CT detection of calcifications in retinoblastoma have a sensitivity of 81–96% and an even higher specificity [24]. Magnetic resonance imaging (MRI) however is currently considered to be of higher accuracy and value due to its superior soft-tissue contrast for determining extent of tumor into orbit, optic nerve, and for evaluation of the presence of pinealoblastoma in trilateral disease. CT scanning is also felt to unnecessarily increase patient exposure to ionizing radiation with limited diagnostic value now that MRI is available. MRI of the brain and orbits with and without contrast is now ordered routinely on all patients with retinoblastoma at the time of diagnosis. The general practice among groups in the United States is to repeat imaging every 6–12 months for germline cases until the age of 5–6 years old to screen to pineal tumors. Transaxial or sagittal T1-weighted images will reveal an RB tumor which is slightly hyperintense with respect to the vitreous body. Transaxial or sagittal heavily T2-weighted imaging provides a low signal intensity of retinoblastoma and is helpful for detecting retinal detachment. Transaxial and sagittal oblique contrast enhanced T11 weighted spin echo provides information of the enhancement of retinal, invasive optic nerve, invasive eye wall, and anterior segment lesions.

2.6.3.7 Genetic counseling

After all of the steps outlined in this chapter are followed, and a diagnosis of retinoblastoma is made, the clinician can hold a discussion with the family regarding therapeutic options and the genetic counseling needed for the patient and their loved ones. A treatment plan can be devised and initiated, but is outside the scope of this chapter, and will be covered in other portions of this text.

3. Conclusion

Accurate and consistent diagnosis of retinoblastoma, and it's simulating lesions begin with the initial consult. This involves a systematic approach starting with a detailed history and high level of suspicion for patients presenting with leukocoria, decreased vision, strabismus, periorbital swelling, or dysmorphic facial features. Initial examination should involve a detailed dilated fundus exam with ophthalmic ultrasound, which will either push the clinician towards or away from the diagnosis of retinoblastoma. Any suspicion should warrant an examination under anesthesia as outlined above to obtain all of the information needed for an accurate diagnosis. The examination under anesthesia should follow a consistent, careful, and repeatable fashion as described earlier in the chapter. The techniques above, if followed, should aid the clinician in consistent diagnosis of retinoblastoma and its simulating lesions. Once diagnosed, appropriate brain and body imaging, and referral for genetic counseling should be performed. Treatment of this rare condition, along with survival and preservation of the eye is continuing to improve and will be covered in other portions of this text.

Acknowledgements

The authors would like to thank David McMahon for his assistance in obtaining many of the photographs used in this chapter.

Conflict of interest

The authors have no conflicts of interests to declare in the production of this book chapter.

Author details

Spencer T. Langevin and Brian P. Marr*
Harkness Eye Institute Columbia University, New York, NY, USA

*Address all correspondence to: bpm2133@cumc.columbia.edu

References

[1] Pawius P. Observationed anatomical. Cited by Bartolini. Bartolini Hafniae. 1657;**16**:336

[2] Kivela T. 200 year of success initiated by James Wardrop's 1809 monograph on retinoblastoma. Acta Ophthalmologica. 2009;**87**:810-812

[3] Stevens A. Case Report. Medical & Surgical, Register. New York: Collins & Co; 1818:117

[4] Wardrop J. Observations on Fungus Haematodes or Soft Cancer. Edinburgh: George Ramsey & Co; 1809. p. 213

[5] Virchow R. Die Krankehaften Geschwulste. Vol. 2. Berlin: August Hirshwald; 1864. pp. 151-169

[6] Hirschberg J. Die Markschwann Die Natzhaut. Berlin: Hirschwald; 1869:3

[7] Flexner S. A peculiar glioma (neuroepithelioma?) of the retina. Bulletin of the Johns Hopkins Hospital. 1891;**2**:115-119

[8] Wintersteiner H. Das Neuroepithelioma Retinae: Eine Anatomisfche Und Klinsche Studie. Vienna: Franz Deuticke; 1897:12-16

[9] Verhoeff FH, Jackson E. Minutes of the proceedings, 62nd annual meeting. Transactions of the American Ophthalmological Society. 1926;**24**:38-43

[10] Maki JL, Marr BP, Abramson DH. Diagnosis of retinoblstoma: How good are referring physicians? Ophthalmic Genetics. 2009;**30**(4):199-205

[11] Grossniklaus HE. Retinoblastoma. Fifty years of progress: The LXXI Edward Jackson memorial lecture. American Journal of Ophthalmology. 2014;**158**(8):875-891

[12] Shields JA, Augsburger JJ. Current approaches to the diagnosis and management of retinoblastoma. Survey of Ophthalmology. 2014;**25**(6):347-372

[13] Gallie BL, Ellsworth RM, Abramson DH, Philips RA. Retinoma: Spontaneous regression of retinoblastoma or benign manifestation of the mutation? British Journal of Cancer. 1982;**45**:513-521

[14] de Graaf P, Göricke S, Rodjan F, Galluzzi P, Maeder P, Castelijns JA, et al. Guidelines for imaging retinoblastoma: Imaging principles and MRI standardization. Pediatric Radiology. 2012;**42**:2-14

[15] Basel A, Bajic D. Preoperative evaluation of the pediatric patient. Anesthesiology Clinics. 2018;**36**:689-700

[16] Lin BA, Messieha ZS, Hoffman WE. Safety and efficacy of pediatric general anesthesia by laryngeal mask airway without intravenous access. International Journal of Clinical Medicine. 2011;**2**:328-331

[17] Quelin C, Bendavid C, Dubourg C, de la Rochebrochard C, Lucas J, Henry C, et al. Twelve new patents with 13q deletion syndrome: Genotype-phenotype analyses in progress. European Journal of Medical Genetics. 2009;**52**:41-46

[18] Shields CL, Shields JA, Baez K, Carter JR, De Potter P. Optic nerve invasion of retinoblastoma; metastatic potential and clinical risk factors. Cancer. 1994;**73**(3):692-698

[19] Kim JW, Ngai LK, Sadda S, Murakami Y, Lee DK, Murphree AL. Retcam fluorescein angiograhy findings in eyes with advanced retinoblastoma. The British Journal of Ophthalmology. 2014;**98**:1666-1671

[20] Sterns GK, Coleman DJ, Ellsworth RM. Characterization and evaluation of retinoblastoma by ultrasonography. Bibliotheca Ophthalmologica. 1975;**83**:125-129

[21] Abramson DH, Ellsworth RM. Ancillary tests for the diagnosis of retinoblastoma. Bulletin of the New York Academy of Medicine. 1980;**56**:221-231

[22] Liu CY, Jonna G, Francis JH, Marr BP, Abramson DH, Brodie SE. Non-selectivity of ERG reductions in eyes treated for retinoblastoma. Documenta Ophthalmologica. 2014;**128**:12-23

[23] Francis JH, Abramson DH, Marr BP, Brodie SE. Ocular manipulation reduces both ipsilateral and contralateral electroretinograms. Documenta Ophthalmologica. 2013;**227**:113-122

[24] Kamihara J, Bourdeaut F, Foulkes WD, Molenaar JJ, Mosse YP, Nakagawara A, et al. Retinoblastoma and neuroblastoma predisposition and surveillance. Clinical Cancer Research. 2017;**23**(13):e98-e106

Chapter 4

Uses of Radiological Imaging in Retinoblastoma

Fahad Albader and Dalal Fatani

Abstract

Retinoblastoma is the most common primary ocular malignancy in children. Diagnosing retinoblastoma relies mainly on the clinical appearance of the lesion and not on histological description. Although histology still remains the gold standard in evaluation of tumor extension and progression risk factor, a tumor biopsy carries high risk of dissemination and is difficult to obtain. Retinoblastoma has characteristic clinical features of creamy-white mass associated with subretinal fluids and may be accompanied by retinal detachment and vitreous seeding. There are many factors contributing to metastatic risk factors like postlaminar optic nerve infiltration, scleral and choroidal invasion, and peribulbar fat invasion. Ancillary testing is necessary for any patient with a suspected retinoblastoma to assess the dimensions of the tumor as well as the tumor extension. An ultrasonography (B scan) will show the mass dimensions as well as the hyperechoic calcifications, which are commonly present with retinoblastoma. CT scan is not the modality of choice for diagnosis of retinoblastoma in children because of the radiation exposure. Magnetic resonance imaging is considered the examination of choice to assess the tumor extension as it has high soft tissue contrast. The use of MRI changed the accuracy of assessing metastatic risk factors as the results yielded before and after the use of MRI differed. This chapter will address the use of radiological imaging in retinoblastoma defining diagnostic characteristics and identifying parameters of metastatic risk factor assessment. This chapter will also include evidence-based review on the efficacy of radiological imaging of retinoblastoma and its impact on the choice of treatment and disease prognosis.

Keywords: magnetic resonance imaging, retinoblastoma, metastasis, optic nerve invasion, vitreous seeding, retinal detachment, calcification, prognosis

1. Introduction

Retinoblastoma is the most common primary ocular malignancy in children. It is usually unilateral but may be bilateral in one-third of cases. It presents in childhood as leukocoria or acute onset strabismus. Diagnosing retinoblastoma relies mainly on the clinical appearance of the lesion and not on histological description. Although histology still remains the gold standard in evaluation of tumors extension and progression risk factor, a tumor biopsy carries high risk of dissemination and is difficult to obtain. Retinoblastoma has characteristic clinical features of creamy-white mass associated with sub retinal fluids and may be accompanied by retinal detachment. Endophytic tumors grow inwards towards the vitreous cavity which may result in vitreous seeding of the tumor cells. Exophytic tumors grow into the sub retinal space causing progressive retinal detachment and subretinal seeing. There are many factors contributing to metastatic risk factors like post laminar optic nerve infiltration, scleral and choroidal invasion, and peribulbar fat invasion. Ancillary testing is necessary for any patient with a suspected retinoblastoma to assess the dimensions of the tumor as well as the tumor extension.

The main ancillary tests that can be used with retinoblastoma are ultrasound imaging (US), computerized tomography (CT), and magnetic resonance imaging (MRI).

Ultrasonography (B scan) will show the mass dimensions as well the hyper-echoic calcifications which is commonly present with retinoblastoma. These imaging modalities and their uses in retinoblastoma detection will be discussed in this chapter with the main focus on MR imaging.

2. Ultrasonography imaging in retinoblastoma

Ultrasound imaging is a cost-effective widely available modality that is non-invasive and easy to perform. This modality is especially useful in patient when the ocular light-conducting media is opaque. It can detect tumor dimensions and characteristics as well as vitreous seeding. It is usually conducted at a 10 MHz high frequency probe. B scans can also visual the optic nerve which can be seen within the retrobulbar fat. The optic nerve is usually seen as a hypoechoic structure within the echogenic surrounding fat.

In case of retinoblastoma, the tumor is visualized as a hyperechoic tumor with irregular borders. It may present a diffuse lesion or a localized well-defined lesion (**Figure 1**). The calcium deposits are clearly visualized by ultrasonography as highly hyper-echoic and they are a pathognomonic feature [1]. Ultrasound imaging can also identify any associated retinal detachment or choroidal thickening (**Figure 2**). The vitreous surrounding the lesion may show hyper-reflective particles representing the calcified tumor seeding into the vitreous cavity.

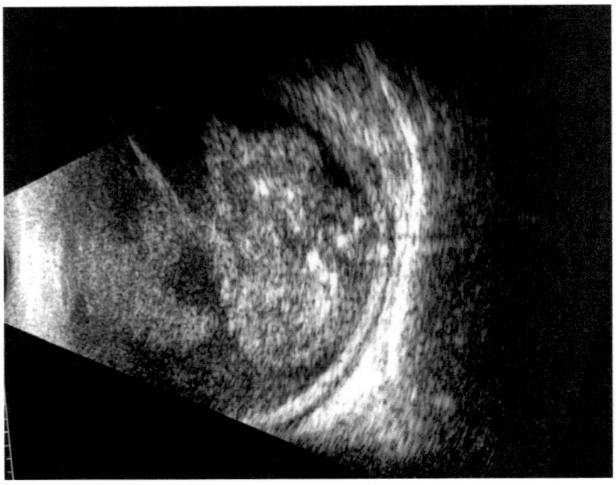

Figure 1.
B scan of an eye with diffuse pattern retinoblastoma showing areas of calcification.

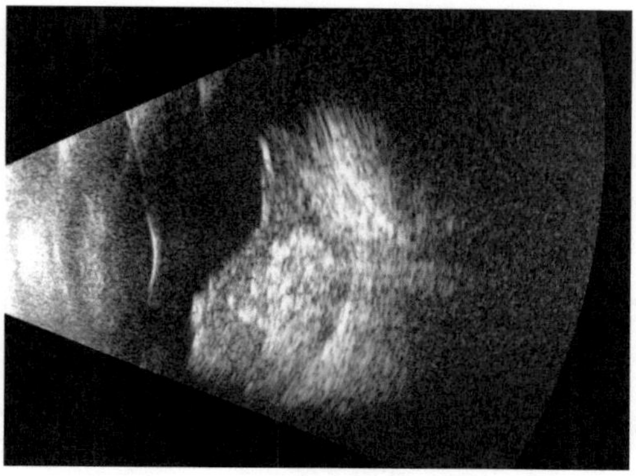

Figure 2.
B scan of an eye with retinoblastoma showing an exophytic growth pattern with an associated retinal detachment.

Extraocular invasion of the optic nerve can also be detected once the normal tubular hypo-echoic nature of it is altered.

3. Computerized tomography imaging in retinoblastoma

Computerized tomography (CT) is a combination of multiple X-ray images from different angles producing cross sectional images. Like standard X-ray, CT depends on relative the radio-density of different tissue structures. CT delivers ionization radiation reaching to 1–10 mSv per brain CT. Retinoblastoma appears as a hyperdense lesion on CT in relation to the surrounding hypodense ocular vitreous (**Figure 3**).

CT scan is also another beneficial tool in detecting calcification which may be seen in a non-homogenous pattern in most large tumors (**Figure 4**) or in a homogenous pattern in smaller tumors. In certain studies, CT scan has failed to show calcification in small retinoblastoma tumors [2–4] CT images can also be useful to detect any associated metastatic brain lesions (**Figure 5**).

CT scan is not the modality of choice for diagnosis and follow-up of children with retinoblastoma due to radiation exposure (ionizing radiation) and the high sensitivity of MRI for soft tissue. This reduces the implantation of CT in retinoblastoma cases especially in areas where MR studies are accessible [3].

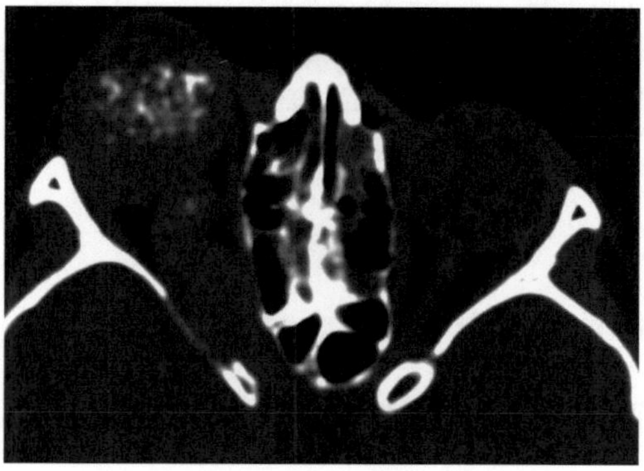

Figure 3.
CT (soft tissue window image) showing right globe hyperdense vitreous, retrolental intraocular solid mass with dystrophic calcification and proximal calcified optic nerve local invasion.

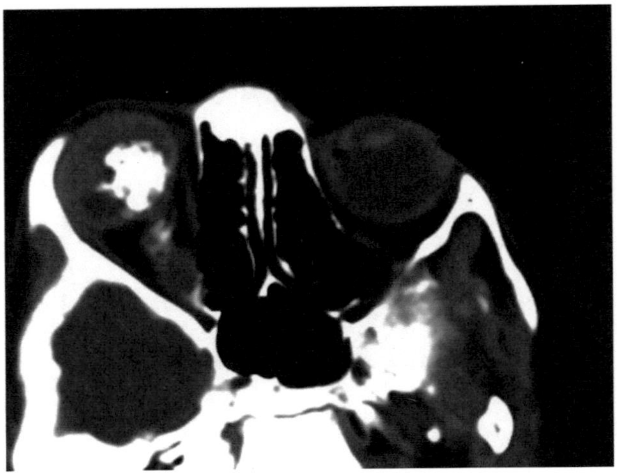

Figure 4.
CT (bone window image) showing right globe enlargement, hyperdense vitreous due to hemorrhage, retrolental intraocular solid mass with central large dystrophic calcification and an enlarged proximal calcified optic nerve due to local invasion.

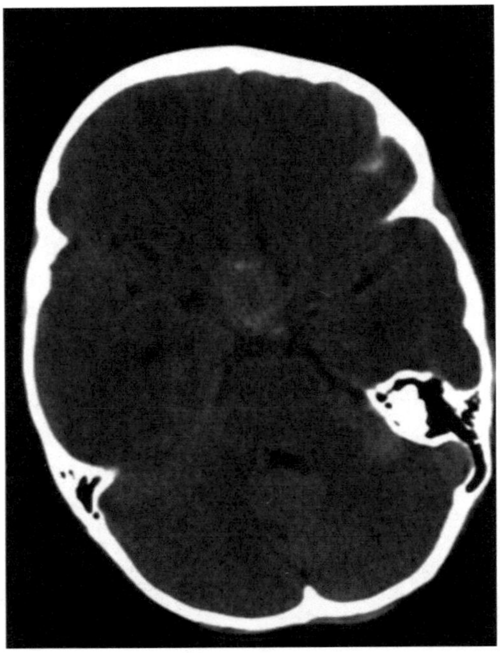

Figure 5.
A non-contrast brain CT for follow up of retinoblastoma patient, showed solid suprasellar mass with faint calcification suggestive of metastasis.

4. Magnetic resonance imaging in retinoblastoma

Magnetic resonance imaging is a type of imaging that use strong magnetic fields and magnetic field gradients to generate anatomical images without the use of ionization radiation.

Magnetic resonance imaging is considered the examination of choice to assess the retinoblastoma tumor extension extraocularly as it has high soft tissue contrast. Although retinoblastoma is usually diagnosed clinically by fundoscopy examination; in cases of unclear ocular medium, MRI can even be used in diagnosing retinoblastoma.

The European Retinoblastoma Imaging Collaboration (ERIC) released a recommended guideline protocol for MR imaging in retinoblastoma. This MR retinoblastoma protocol uses a 1.5 T in T_1 weighted images scout view and turbo spin-echo T_2 and PD images if the brain as well as 2 mm thick T_2 images of the eye in sagittal cuts. Later axial T_1 images and T_2 with fat suppression of the orbit with contrast medium of 0.1 mmol/kg gadopentetate dimeglumine are obtained. The advanced use of high resolution three-dimensional T_2 weighted imaging allows for then 0.4 mm sections with high SNR that is sensitive to detect calcification.

In this guideline a post laminar optic nerve invasion is characterized by abnormal contrast enhancement of the optic nerve that is > = 2 mm length or any asymmetrical thickening [5].

Sagittal and axial T_1-weighted images: repetition time (TR) = 475 ms; echo time (TE) = 10 ms; slice thickness = 2 mm; field of view (FOV) = 150 × 150 mm; matrix = 256 × 179; number of excitations = 1].

Axial T_2-weighted fat sat images: TR = 3600 ms; TE = 95 ms; echo train length = 15; slice thickness = 2.5 mm; FOV = 150 × 150 mm; matrix = 320 × 240; number of excitations = 2].

When approaching MRI images of an intraocular lesion, one of the first parameters to be assessed is the axial length and eye volume as well as the laterality of the disease. Thorough examination of the brain images is also a major step for the detection of any syndromic associations or intracranial metastasis. These parameters are very beneficial in the differentiation of similar intraocular lesions. In cases of persistent fetal vasculature (PFV), they can present with leukocoria or strabismus as well. However, the globe size is markedly smaller in PFV cases (**Figure 6**).

On MRI the retinoblastoma tumor borders usually exhibit an irregular lobulated pattern.

The eye parameters are relatively smaller in eyes with retinoblastoma with the size of the tumor volume inversely proportional to the size of the globe [6].

Retinoblastoma can also be associated with retinal detachment which can be clearly detectable on MR images (**Figure 7**).

Retinoblastoma on T_1 weighted MR imaging appears as relatively hyper-intense compared to the adjacent normal vitreous. It also contains areas of low signal intensity within the hyper-intense tumor that reflects the areas of calcification (**Figure 8**).

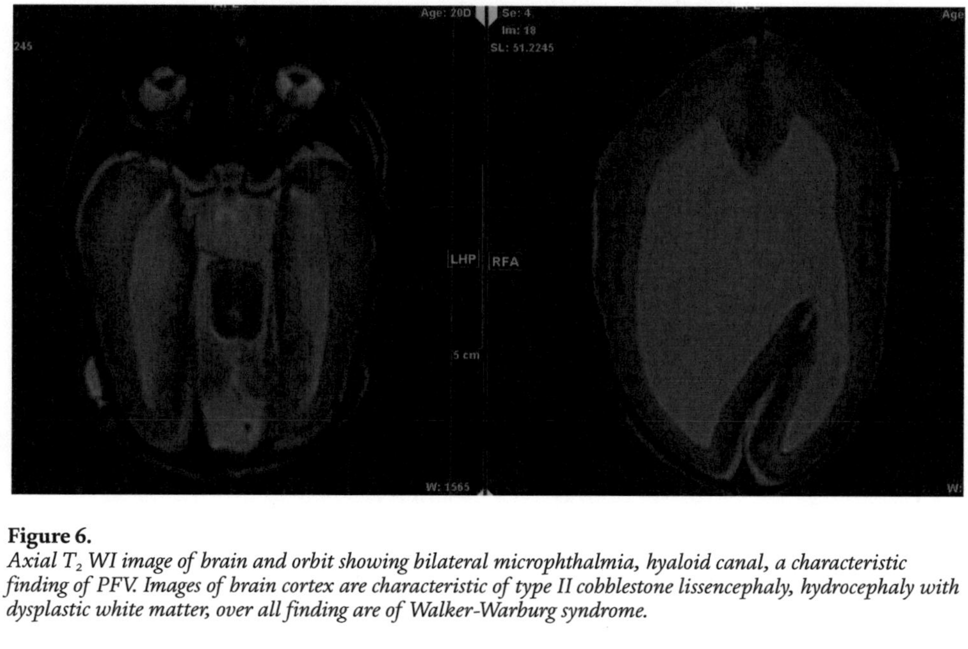

Figure 6.
Axial T_2 WI image of brain and orbit showing bilateral microphthalmia, hyaloid canal, a characteristic finding of PFV. Images of brain cortex are characteristic of type II cobblestone lissencephaly, hydrocephaly with dysplastic white matter, over all finding are of Walker-Warburg syndrome.

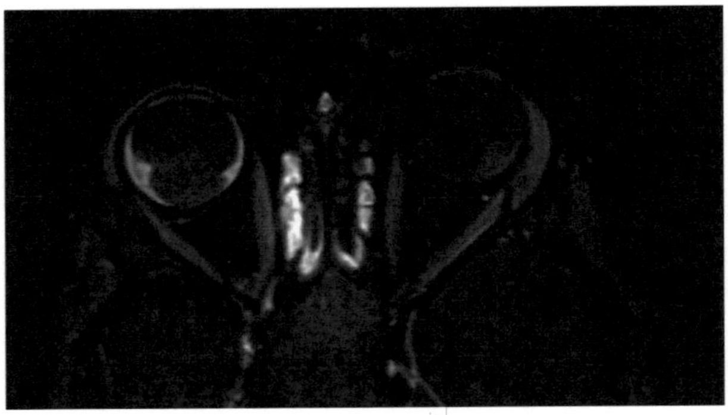

Figure 7.
MRI orbit T_1 weighted fat saturated with contrast imaging showing bilateral faintly enhanced retrolental retinal based mass with right retinal detachment.

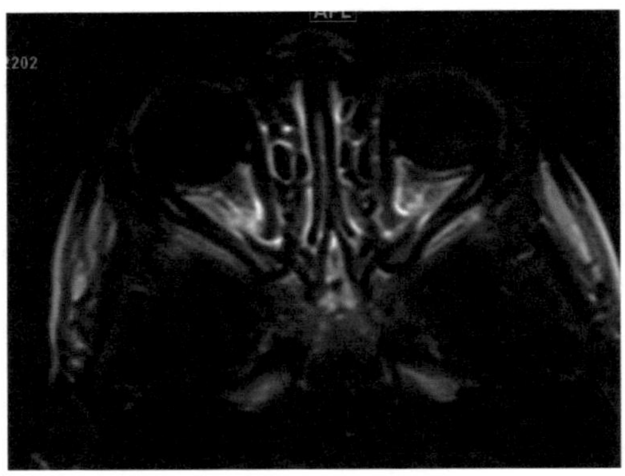

Figure 8.
MRI T_1 weighted image with contrast, faintly enhanced retrolental mass at left globe corresponding to retinoblastoma tumor core.

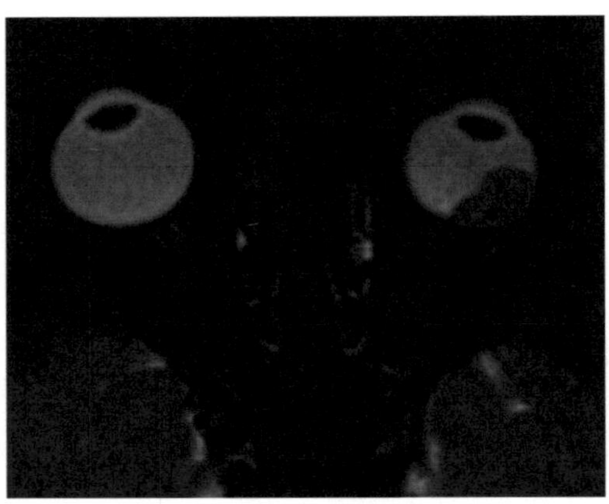

Figure 9.
MRI T_2 weighted fat saturated image of the orbits showing low signal of retrolental mass corresponding to retinoblastoma tumor at left globe with mild reduction of size of globe.

A study compared the efficacy of MRI in calcification detection by comparing in vivo T_2 weight MRI with ex vivo high-resolution CT. It has found the T_2WI correlated well with CT findings. Therefore, combining examination with

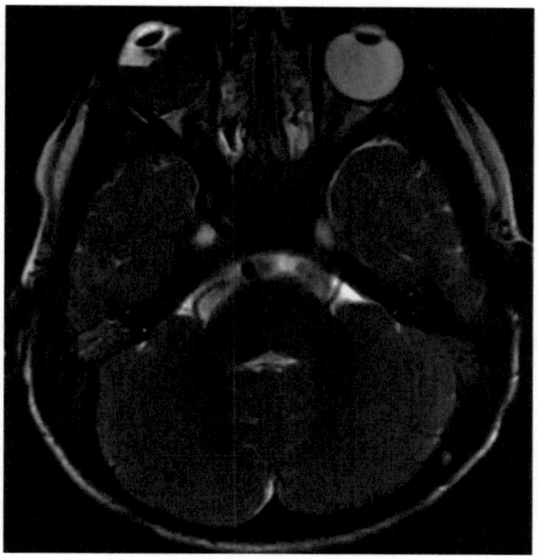

Figure 10.
Axial T_2 weighed MRI of the brain and orbit showing a hypointense tumor of the right globe, filling 80% if the globe with areas of hypo-intensity representing calcification or retinoblastoma tumor core.

ultrasonography and MRI with gradient-echo sequence is thought to be the standard diagnostic approach for any patient with retinoblastoma [4].

On T_2 weighted imaging, the retinoblastoma tumor is usually darker than the vitreous resulting in a relative hypo-intense lesion within the vitreous with further patches of hypointensity within corresponding to calcification area (**Figures 9** and **10**).

5. Diffusion weighted imaging in retinoblastoma

Diffusion-weighted imaging (DWI) is a type of MR imaging that depends on the motion of water molecule within the tissue. Highly cellular tissue exhibits lower diffusion coefficients making this modality useful for tumor characterization. DWI is wisely wised for orbital disease as well as brain malignancy. On diffusion weighted imaging (*P* value 1000) the retinoblastoma tumor shows diffuse restriction.

A pulse sequence form of DWI that generates various imaging is referred to as ADC images (apparent diffusion coefficient) which measures the magnitude of diffusion resulting a numerical value. The mean ADC value of retinoblastoma was $0.49 \pm 0.12 \times 10^{-3}$ mm^2/s.

The low ADC values of retinoblastoma tumors are attributed to the tightly packed nature of high nuclear cytoplasmic ratio of the tumor (**Figure 11**).

The use of ADC value images has shown to be well correlated with the degree of tumor differentiation in a study conducted in Saudi Arabia. The ADC value was analyzed in different sized tumors and was shown to be significantly different with various sized tumors. It demonstrates an inverse correlation of the ADC value with the tumor size. The ADC value of small tumors (<10 mm) was $0.55 \pm 0.09 \times 10^{-3}$ mm^2/s, medium tumors (>10–15 mm) was $0.48 \pm 0.09 \times 10^{-3}$ mm^2/s, and large tumors (>15 mm) was of $0.38 \pm 0.11 \times 10^{-3}$ mm^2/s value.

In addition, the ADC value was lower in tumors with optic nerve invasion which may correlate with the tumor's likelihood to be poorly differentiated and

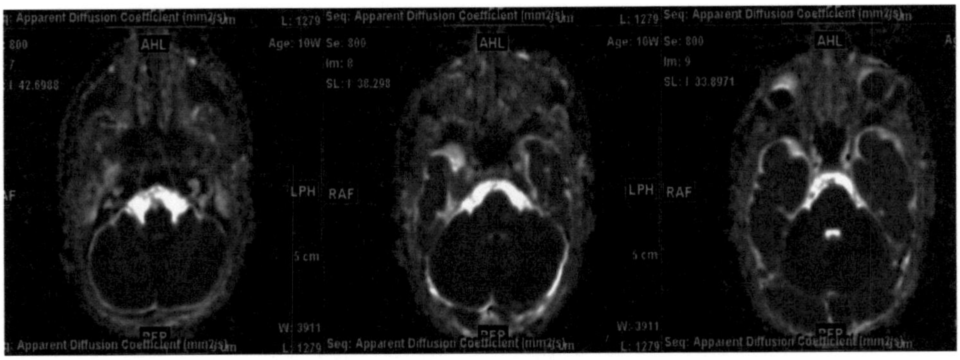

Figure 11.
ADC (apparent diffusion coefficient) MR image of the brain and orbit showing bilateral ocular lesions with low ADC values represented tumor core representing bilateral retinoblastoma.

aggressive [7]. *Axial diffusion weighted images: TR = 5000 ms; TE = 74 ms; number of diffusion matrix = 200 – 162; number of excitations = 1 with reconstruction of the ADC map.*

6. Metastasis of retinoblastoma on MRI

Retinoblastoma tumor grows with an endophytic and/or an exophytic pattern. Endophytic growth starts from the inner layers of the retina progressing into the vitreous cavity. As the tumor cells detach from the main tumor, they can float into the vitreous and cause what is known as vitreous seeding. Detection of vitreous seeding is crucial in the staging of retinoblastoma and is considered a main prognostic indicator. Although detection of vitreous seeding by ophthalmoscopy examination is superior to MR imaging, it can be clearly identified in 63% of patient on MRI. It is usually identified as bright patches on T_1 weighted imaging and dark patches on T_2 weighted imaging within the vitreous cavity [5, 8] (**Figure 12**).

Exophytic growth pattern starts at the outer retinal layers and progress into the sub-retinal space causing a retinal detachment and sub-retinal tumor seeding [9].

MR imaging can detect choroidal invasion of retinoblastoma tumor at a sensitivity of 74% and a specificity of 72%. (Brisse relevance) Scleral invasion of retinoblastoma tumor can also be assessed by MR imaging with 88% sensitivity and 99% specificity [2] (**Figure** 7).

Another more aggressive pattern of retinoblastoma tumor growth is diffuse infiltrating growth pattern. In this pattern, the tumor grows along the retina as a placoid mass which subsequently results in ocular inflammation and hemorrhages. This may be seen as severe AS inflammation and a pseudohypopyon. MR images can help assess the anterior segment for the presenter absence if abnormal enhancement.

Diffuse infiltrative growth pattern is very rare (1–2%) and occurs with older age children with a male predilection of 8:1. It is usually difficult to diagnose as there are no discrete mass borders and it usually lacks the characteristic retinoblastoma calcification. A retinal detachment is commonly associated and is often evident on MRI especially on FLAIR sequence (Fluid attenuated inversion recovery) [10].

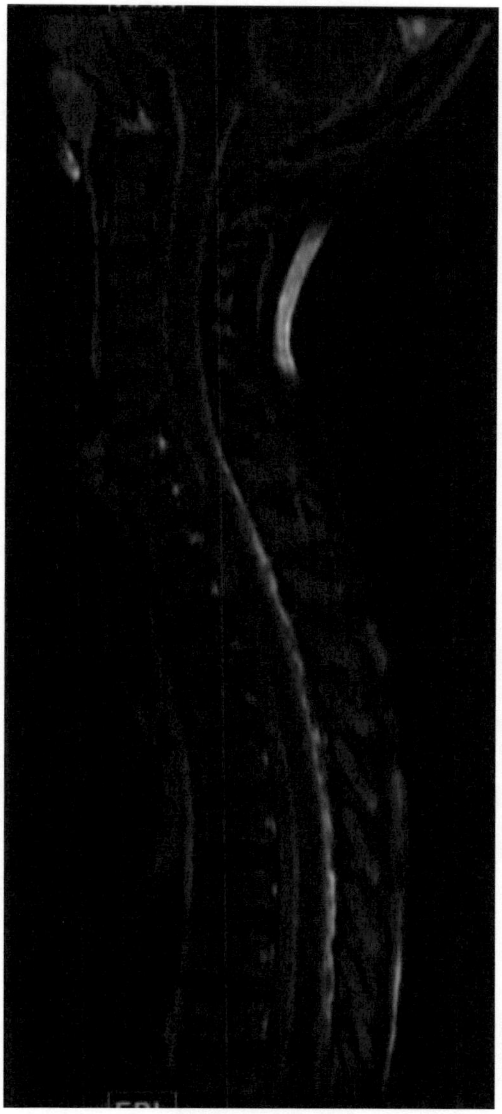

Figure 12.
MRI of the spine showing areas of diffuse leptomeningeal enhancement of the spinal cord representing areas of CSF seeding.

7. MRI's uses in the staging and prognosis of retinoblastoma

Although MRI can aid in the diagnosis of retinoblastoma by the aforementioned characteristics, it is more widely used for the staging of retinoblastoma. Like all other malignancies, tumor staging in retinoblastoma is essential for the prognosis predictions.

The use of MRI has changed the accuracy of assessing metastatic risk factors as the initial retinoblastoma staging of patients before the use of MRI varied after MR imaging were obtained.

The extension of retinoblastoma is usually by direct extension into adjacent structures. Intraocular extension of the tumor can easily be visualized during examination in patients with good posterior pole visualization. MR imaging has been widely used to evaluate the extra-ocular and intracranial extension and can also aid in the evaluation of intraocular tumor extension [11].

Intraocular extension can be detected by choroidal irregularities. Choroidal invasion identification is important in the prognosis of the disease. It changes the prognosis of retinoblastoma by increasing the mortality rate up to 24–65% depending on the severity of invasion [12].

In the assessment of extra-ocular retinoblastoma extension, the most important structure to evaluate is the optic nerve. Involvement of the optic nerve in retinoblastoma alters the prognosis and the management of the disease. The overall mortality rate of retinoblastoma without optic nerve invasion is 10%. If the invasion of the optic nerve reaches through the lamina cribrosa, the mortality may rise up to 15%. Moreover, if the extension is posterior to the lamina cribrosa the mortality rises up to 44%. This makes the optic nerve assessment by MR imaging crucial in any retinoblastoma case with proper identification of the level of optic nerve invasion. On MRI, the affected optic nerve appears thickened and irregular with high enhancement of the nerve itself and the area surrounding it [11].

A study showed that the specificity of MRI in detecting optic nerve invasion past the lamina cribrosa to reach up to 80% and a sensitivity of 74%. This makes MR imaging the most superior non-invasive method in the detection of retinoblastoma optic nerve invasion [13] (**Figures 13** and **14**).

Ophthalmic surgeons require extra measurements of the invasion to take extra precautions during the enucleation of the affected eye. It is important for the MR image to demonstrate if the retrolaminar optic nerve invasion extends more than 5 mm posteriorly. This is particularly crucial to identify prior to surgical intervention as the tumor may be cut through during the enucleation. If such complication happens, the distal part of the tumor that remains is connected to the brain and may progress to brain metastasis. In such cases, the surgeon might consider doing an orbitotomy to be able to reach further posterior and dissect at least 10 mm from

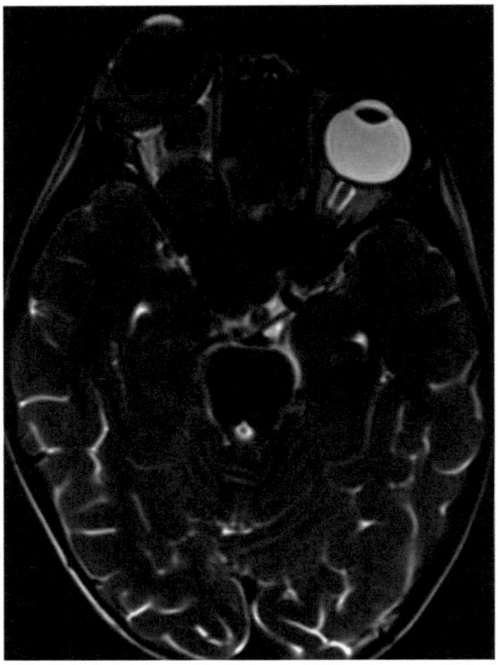

Figure 13.
MRI T_2 weighted image of brain and orbit showing right globe retrolental hypo-intense tumor core, retro bulbar extension and extensive long segment right optic nerve invasion resulting in right globe proptosis.

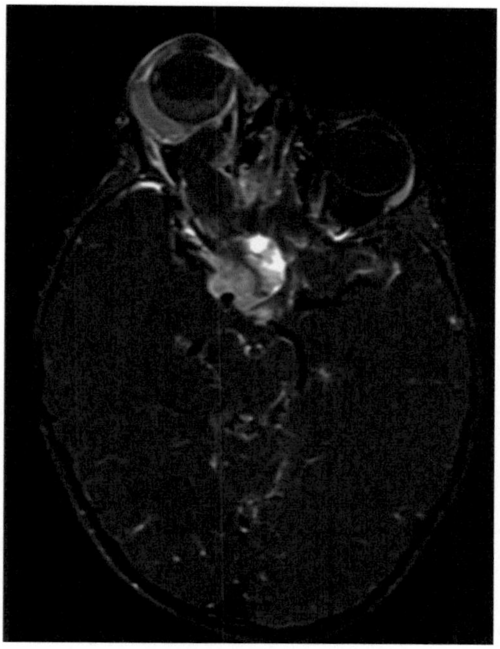

Figure 14.
MRI T_1 weighted image with contrast of the same patient delineating the retrobulbar extension, enhanced and enlarged right optic nerve, leptomeningeal enhancement due to direct extension and CSF seeding of retinoblastoma.

the suggested tumor margin. Despite the advancement of MRI, it has limitations in detecting microscopic optic nerve invasion. Studies have shown a discrepancy between histological results in optic nerve assessment (gold standard) and MRI results [14]. This dictates the need for thorough histopathological assessment of the optic nerve regardless of MR findings.

An important disease entity in retinoblastoma is the trilateral retinoblastoma disease. It refers to rare disease that is characterized by bilateral ocular RB and a primitive midline neuroectodermal tumor in the pineal region or the suprasellar cistern. It represents 1.5–5% of all RB patients [15].

8. Conclusion

Retinoblastoma is the most common primary ocular malignancy in children. Diagnostic imaging has changed the accuracy of diagnosing and staging retinoblastoma. There are many imaging modalities that are currently in use for retinoblastoma tumor like ultrasonography, computerized tomography and magnetic resonance imaging. MR images of the brain and spinal cord need to be obtained routinely in retinoblastoma patients in institutes where MRI is accessible. They aid in the diagnosis and prognosis of the disease. As the retinoblastoma tumor seeding may spread via cerebrospinal fluid and reach the intracranial resulting in brain metastasis, MRI can clearly delineate these metastatic lesions, which eventually alters the management plan.

MRI can show retrolaminar optic nerve and choroidoscleral infiltration and spread of tumor into the brain and spine more accurately than other diagnostic imaging.

A purely ocular tumor confined within the globe reaches a survival rate of 90% AT 5-years whereas a tumor that has extended outside the globe has a mortality rate of over 90%.

This drastic difference makes staging and the use of ancillary testing vital for the prognosis and survival rate estimation which further guides the treatment decision.

It is now currently recommended for any newly diagnosed patient with retinoblastoma to undergo an MRI [13].

MRI can also offer hope for future advancement of early diagnosis. It has recently shown to aid in very early fetal diagnosis of retinoblastoma in a fetus with high-risk of RB and may be implemented as a part of future screening protocol in high risk population [16].

Acknowledgements

The authors would like to thank King Khaled University Hospital and King Abdulaziz University Hospital under the King Saud University Institute for the images provided.

Conflict of interest

There is no financial interest to disclose.

Author details

Fahad Albader and Dalal Fatani*
King Saud University, Riyadh, Saudi Arabia

*Address all correspondence to: dalal.fatani@gmail.com

References

[1] Aironi VD, Gandage SG. Pictorial essay: B-scan ultrasonography in ocular abnormalities. Indian Journal of Radiology and Imaging. 2009;**19**(2):109-115

[2] Arrigg PG, Hedges TR 3rd, Char DH. Computed tomography in the diagnosis of retinoblastoma. British Journal of Ophthalmology. 1983;**67**(9):588-591

[3] de Jong MC, de Graaf P, Noij DP, Goricke S, Maeder P, Galluzzi P, et al. Diagnostic performance of magnetic resonance imaging and computed tomography for advanced retinoblastoma: A systematic review and meta-analysis. Ophthalmology. 2014;**121**(5):1109-1118

[4] Rodjan F, de Graaf P, van der Valk P, Hadjistilianou T, Cerase A, Toti P, et al. Detection of calcifications in retinoblastoma using gradient-echo MR imaging sequences: Comparative study between in vivo MR imaging and ex vivo high-resolution CT. American Journal of Neuroradiology. 2015;**36**(2):355-360

[5] de Graaf P, Goricke S, Rodjan F, Galluzzi P, Maeder P, Castelijns JA, et al. Guidelines for imaging retinoblastoma: Imaging principles and MRI standardization. Pediatric Radiology. 2012;**42**(1):2-14

[6] de Graaf P, Knol DL, Moll AC, Imhof SM, Schouten-van Meeteren AY, Castelijns JA. Eye size in retinoblastoma: MR imaging measurements in normal and affected eyes. Radiology. 2007;**244**(1):273-280

[7] Abdel Razek AA, Elkhamary S, Al-Mesfer S, Alkatan HM. Correlation of apparent diffusion coefficient at 3T with prognostic parameters of retinoblastoma. American Journal of Neuroradiology. 2012;**33**(5):944-948

[8] Lemke AJ, Kazi I, Mergner U, Foerster PI, Heimann H, Bechrakis N, et al. Retinoblastoma—MR appearance using a surface coil in comparison with histopathological results. European Radiology. 2007;**17**(1):49-60

[9] de Graaf P, Barkhof F, Moll AC, Imhof SM, Knol DL, van der Valk P, et al. Retinoblastoma: MR imaging parameters in detection of tumor extent. Radiology. 2005;**235**(1):197-207

[10] Brisse HJ, Lumbroso L, Freneaux PC, Validire P, Doz FP, Quintana EJ, et al. Sonographic, CT, and MR imaging findings in diffuse infiltrative retinoblastoma: Report of two cases with histologic comparison. American Journal of Neuroradiology. 2001;**22**(3):499-504

[11] Brisse HJ, Guesmi M, Aerts I, Sastre-Garau X, Savignoni A, Lumbroso-Le Rouic L, et al. Relevance of CT and MRI in retinoblastoma for the diagnosis of postlaminar invasion with normal-size optic nerve: A retrospective study of 150 patients with histological comparison. Pediatric Radiology. 2007;**37**(7):649-656

[12] Galluzzi P, Cerase A, Hadjistilianou T, De Francesco S, Toti P, Vallone IM, et al. Retinoblastoma: Abnormal gadolinium enhancement of anterior segment of eyes at MR imaging with clinical and histopathologic correlation. Radiology. 2003;**228**(3):683-690

[13] Khurana A, Eisenhut CA, Wan W, Ebrahimi KB, Patel C, O'Brien JM, et al. Comparison of the diagnostic value of MR imaging and ophthalmoscopy for the staging of retinoblastoma. European Radiology. 2013;**23**(5):1271-1280

[14] Wilson MW, Rodriguez-Galindo C, Billups C, Haik BG, Laningham F, Patay Z. Lack of correlation between the histologic and magnetic resonance imaging results of optic

nerve involvement in eyes primarily enucleated for retinoblastoma. Ophthalmology. 2009;**116**(8):1558-1563

[15] Provenzale JM, Gururangan S, Klintworth G. Trilateral retinoblastoma: Clinical and radiologic progression. American Journal of Roentgenology. 2004;**183**(2):505-511

[16] Staffieri SE, McGillivray G, Elder JE, Bristowe A, Cole S, McKenzie JD, et al. Managing fetuses at high risk of retinoblastoma: Lesion detection on screening MRI. Prenatal Diagnosis. 2015;**35**(2):174-178

Chapter 5

Retinoblastoma: Update on Current Management

Abdullah Almater, Abdulrahman Alfaleh, Khalid Alshomar and Saleh AlMesfer

Abstract

Retinoblastoma (Rb) is the most common primary intraocular malignancy in children with an incidence from 1:15,000 to 1:20,000 live births. It can present as a unilateral or bilateral involvement of the eyes. It is generally induced by biallelic mutation of the RB1 tumor suppressor gene that leads to malignant transformation of primitive retinal cells. The most common presentation is leukocoria, followed by strabismus. The initial assessment and future treatment of such tumor should be based on the laterality, the stage of the tumor, and the presenting age of the child. In general, the primary target of therapy is to preserve the child's life. However, preserving the globe and preserving vision should be achieved whenever it's possible. Retinoblastoma treatment has evolved from enucleating the affected globe to also involving external beam radiation therapy, cryotherapy, laser photocoagulation, thermotherapy, brachytherapy, and chemotherapy (intravitreal, intra-arterial, and systematic). This chapter is intended to discuss briefly the clinical presentation of Rb, as well as a comprehensive review about the evolution and current treatment modalities with a focus on cases with low-risk features.

Keywords: retinoblastoma, management, enucleation, external beam radiation therapy, brachytherapy, thermotherapy, laser photocoagulation, cryotherapy, chemotherapy

1. Clinical presentation and diagnosis

The clinical presentation of retinoblastoma can be variable depending on the stage of the tumor. However, the most common presenting symptom overall is abnormal white reflection from one or both pupils [1]. This can be observed grossly by the naked eye and is termed as leukocoria. The second most common presentation of retinoblastoma is strabismus, which results from sensory deprivation when the tumor involves the central vision [2]. Less commonly, uveitis, glaucoma, hyphema, iris heterochromia, and orbital cellulitis can also be presenting signs for retinoblastoma [3]. A more advance and late presentation may result in proptosis and orbital swelling [4]. Any of the mentioned clinical presentations in a child should prompt detailed clinical exam including dilated fundus examination. Typically, it shows unifocal or multifocal white vascularized retinal mass with or without tumor seeding. Different imaging modalities can be performed to aid in the diagnoses of retinoblastoma. The most easy and readily available modality is ultrasound. It can be helpful in the detection of intraocular mass characteristic

IntechOpen

(height, thickness, and depth) and the presence of heterogeneity and calcification. Computed tomography (CT) is more sensitive in detecting intraocular calcification and delineating the mass. However, CT scan raises the concern of developing secondary malignancies in cases with germ line mutation due to radiations [5]. Magnetic resonance imaging (MRI) is currently the preferred imaging modality of choice for most ophthalmologists. MRI is considered the best for detecting optic nerve involvement and extraocular extension [6]. Other diagnostic procedures like cerebrospinal fluid (CSF) analysis and cytology are particularly performed when there is evidence of optic nerve involvement grossly or microscopically based on histopathologic examination after enucleation. Bone marrow biopsy is indicated for bone marrow metastasis based on clinical exam or blood work-up. Diagnosis of retinoblastoma should be based on clinical examination that is supported by imaging techniques. However, differentiating retinoblastoma from other conditions like persistent hyperplastic primary vitreous (PHPV), Coats' disease, or toxocariasis can be challenging [7–11]. Different classifications have been proposed for retinoblastoma staging throughout the past decades, including TNMH (tumor, node, metastasis, heritable trait) cancer staging for the American Joint Committee on Cancer (AJCC), Reese-Ellsworth classification system (R-E), and International Intraocular Retinoblastoma Classification (IIRC) [12–16]. The International Intraocular Retinoblastoma Classification or International Classification of Retinoblastoma (ICRB) have been widely accepted by ophthalmologists since they were first introduced in 2003, to predict the outcomes following chemoreduction for retinoblastoma [15, 16] (**Table 1** and **Figure 1**).

Group	Subgroup	Reference	Features
A	Very low risk	Small tumor	• RB ≤3 mm (in basal dimension) • Al least 3 mm away from the foveola and 1.5 mm from the optic nerve • No vitreous or subretinal seeding is present
B	Low risk	Larger tumor Macula Juxtapapillary Subretinal fluid	• RB >3 mm (in basal dimension) • Macular location (≤3 mm to foveola) • Juxtapapillary location (≤1.5 mm to optic nerve) • Additional subretinal fluid (≤3 mm from margin) • No vitreous or subretinal seeding is present
C	Moderate risk	Focal seeds	• Focal subretinal and/or vitreous seeds ≤3 mm from the tumor
D	High risk	Diffuse seeds	• Diffuse subretinal and/or vitreous seeds >3 mm from the tumor
E	Very high risk	Extensive retinoblastoma	• Extensive retinoblastoma occupying >50% of globe or any of the following: • Secondary neovascular glaucoma • Tumor anterior to anterior vitreous face or touching the lens • Diffuse infiltrating retinoblastoma • Massive intraocular hemorrhage • Aseptic orbital cellulitis • Phthisis bulbi

Table 1.
International intraocular retinoblastoma classification.

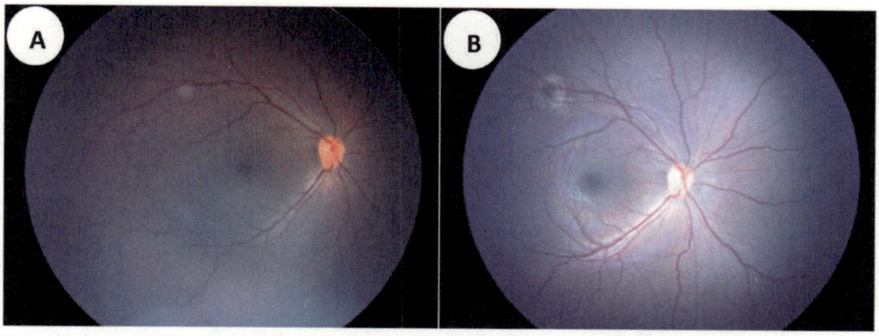

Case 1: One-month-old female with strong family history of retinoblastoma that was diagnosed with unilateral retinoblastoma through family screening program. (A) Showing single active lesion along the continuation of the superior-temporal arcade in the right eye (group A). (B) Showing the same lesion 1-month post-TTT.

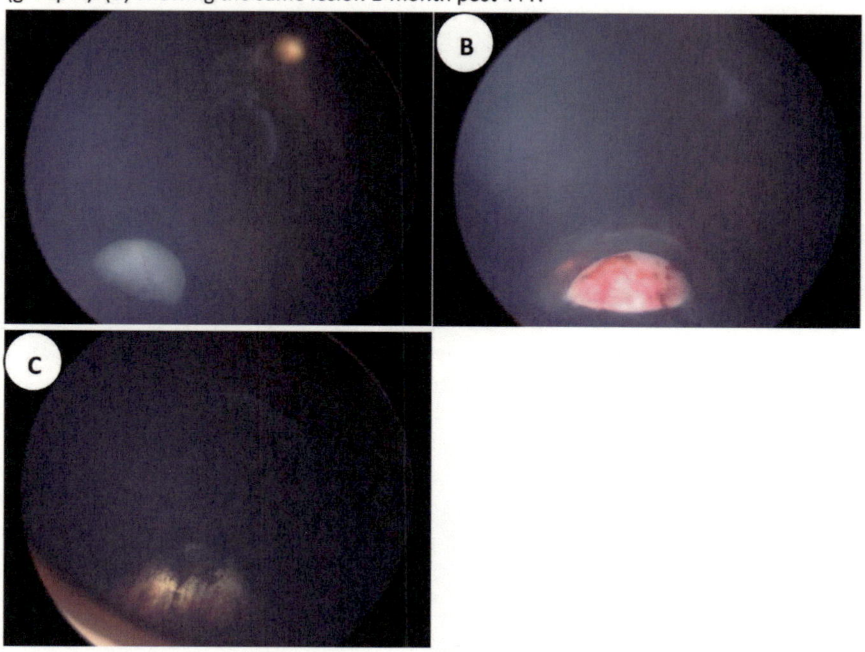

Case 2: Two-year-old male with bilateral retinoblastoma (OD, group E; OS, group A). (A) Single thick whitish lesion located inferior-temporal in the left eye (group A). (B) Same lesion with hemorrhages post-cryotherapy and TTT in the same month. (C) Flat scarred lesion after 3 months. Right eye photos are not shown here.

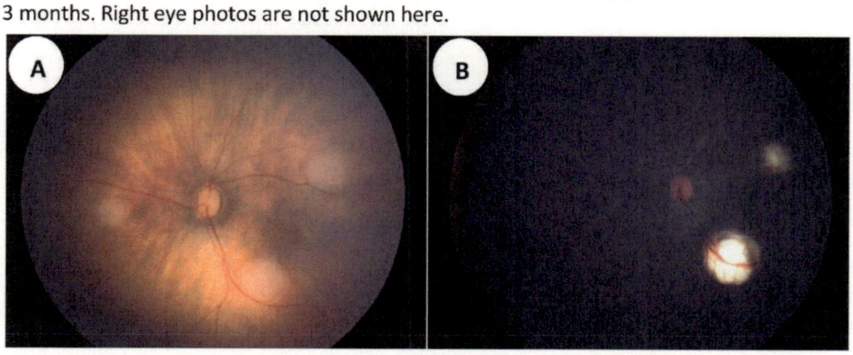

Case 3: Twenty-eight-day-old male diagnosed with bilateral retinoblastoma (group B). (A) Left eye showing three active whitish lesions (one large macular lesion measuring >3 mm in size, two smaller lesions at superior-temporal arcade and inferior-nasal arcade (group B)). (B) Flat and scarred lesions 3 years post-TTT and intravenous chemotherapy. Right eye photos are not shown here.

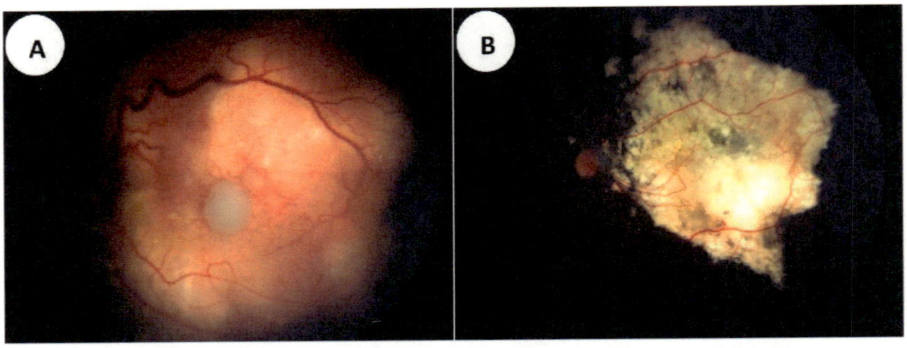

Case 4: Eight-month-old female with unilateral sporadic retinoblastoma. (A) Left eye showing large subretinal macular lesion, with initial subretinal seeding (group C). (B) Similar lesion showing regressing and calcification (cottage cheese appearance) 2 years after multiple TTT and intravenous chemotherapy.

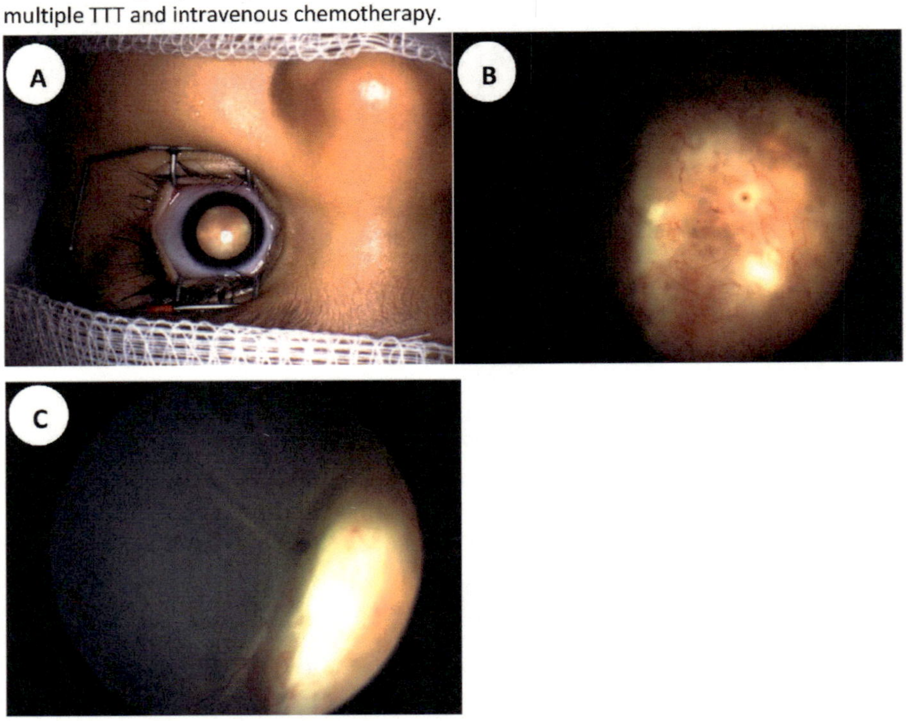

Case 5: Five-month-old male with unilateral retinoblastoma. (A) External photo of the left eye showing leukocoria. (B) Left eye showing large temporal and inferior-temporal lesion with calcification and secondary retinal detachment (group D). (C) Fundus photo showing the secondary serous retinal detachment. Patient underwent enucleation for the left eye.

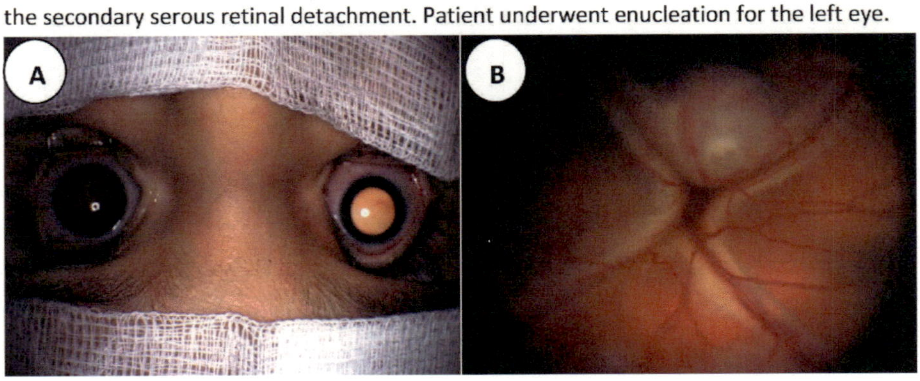

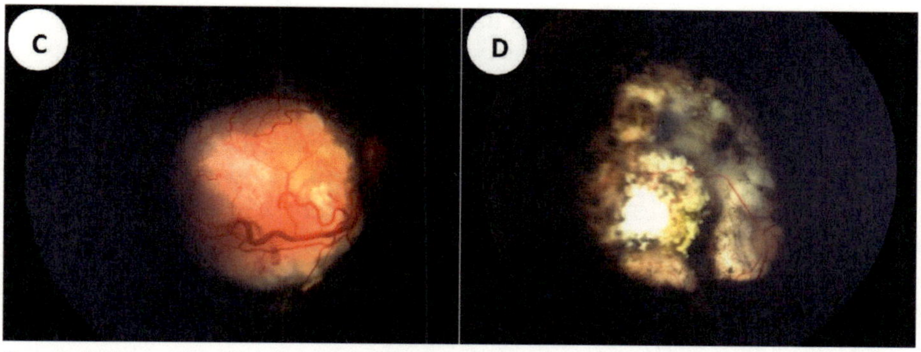

Case 6: Eight-month-old male with bilateral retinoblastoma (OD, group C; OS, group E). (A) External photo of both eyes showing leukocoria in the right eye and dim reflex for the left eye. (B) Fundus photo of the left eye showing large whitish lesion in the posterior pole with total retinal detachment (group E). (C) Right eye showing large vascularized elevated whitish lesion involving the macula. (D) Scarred macular lesion 14 months post-TTT and intravenous chemotherapy. The patient underwent enucleation of the left eye.

Figure 1.
Retinoblastoma tumors, according to the international intraocular retinoblastoma classification, and their response to treatments.

2. Management

Management of retinoblastoma is complex and requires a multidisciplinary team approach that includes an ophthalmologist, pediatric oncologist, radiation oncologist, pathologist, geneticist, social worker, nurses, and others. The primary goal of treatment is to save the child's life and then to salvage the globe and optimize the vision if possible. A multimodal therapeutic option for retinoblastoma is available, which ranges from focal therapies like laser photocoagulation, cryotherapy, thermotherapy, and plaque radiotherapy to enucleation or chemotherapy for more advance cases. The decision for choosing a treatment option is depending on several factors including the laterality, tumor size and histopathologic feature, the age and general health of the child, and the family desires.

3. Enucleation

Enucleation is the preferred option for most children presenting with advance tumor (group E eyes), especially if unilateral [17–21]. Other indications for enucleation are failure of all possible effective therapies, active tumor in an eye with no visual potential, anterior segment invasion, secondary neovascular glaucoma, and when the visualization of the tumor is compromised due to corneal opacity, cataract, or vitreous hemorrhage [22]. Enucleation is rarely indicated for bilateral retinoblastoma due to devastating functional limitation that follows such decision. The goal during enucleation is to obtain as much optic nerve as possible (usually 8–12 mm) to make sure that the surgical margin is free from tumor [23, 24]. Surgeons should avoid perforation of the globe during the procedure to minimize the potential risk of tumor seeding into the orbital tissue [25]. Histopathologic evaluation post enucleation allows for evaluation of high-risk features that requires additional chemotherapy. These features include retrolaminar optic nerve invasion, choroidal invasion, scleral and orbital invasion, and anterior chamber seeding [26–28]. At the time of enucleation, an orbital implant is placed to ensure proper growth of the orbit and allows for free movement of the prosthesis when attaching the extraocular muscles to the implant [4, 29]. Many different orbital implants can used and are generally divided to porous and nonporous implants. The most commonly used are porous implants, hence allowing vascular growth in the tiny pores within the implant. This can serve in the stabilization of the implant while minimizing the risk of exposure and extrusion or infection [4, 25].

4. External beam radiation therapy (EBRT)

External beam radiation therapy is an important modality used in the treatment of retinoblastoma. However, due to serious adverse effects, it has fallen out of use and became preserved for moderately advanced disease where retinoblastoma is refractory or progressive after chemotherapy to salvage the eye from enucleation. EBRT techniques have improved overtime, and new methods aim to eliminate the disease and minimize normal tissue exposure to avoid any adverse effects [30–33].

The main EBRT techniques used in treating retinoblastoma are photon or electron radiation therapy (ERT), intensity-modulated radiation therapy (IMRT), and proton radiation therapy (PRT). IMRT and PRT allow for more conformal radiotherapy options in addition to a unique physical property of PRT. Rather than traversing the target, protons stops at energy-dependent depth and with a reduced exit dose to almost zero where it reduces the injury to uninvolved structures and limit the radiation beams to a specific area. This physical property has shown to decrease unwanted adverse effects, making PRT become superior to photon therapy [30, 31].

EBRT treatment sessions are usually scheduled over a period of weeks where multiple small fractions of radiation are delivered via an external machine targeting the lesion. This increases tumor sensitivity to radiation by allowing time for reoxygenation and reassortment of cell cycle. It also spares normal tissues by allowing time for repair in between fractions. Conversely, PRT is delivered in one or a few large fractions, but to small discrete volumes, hence minimizing the volume of surrounding irradiated normal tissue [30, 34].

The outcome of patients who were treated with EBRT has been studied over the past decades. Enucleation was ultimately required in 18–37.5% of eyes, and local failure after radiotherapy was similar between PRT and ERT. Vision was preserved in most of the cases with an outcome showing up to 70% of patients having no or mild visual impairment. Moderate visual impairment is seen in 10–23% of eyes, whereas poor or no useful vision was in 20–41.7% of non-enucleated eyes. The best visual outcomes are noted in patients with early stages that spared the optic disc, macula, and fovea, suggesting that the location of tumors has an impact of visual outcome even after PRT [35–38].

Acute toxicities that can be seen after therapy sessions include local erythema of the skin, hyperpigmentation, erythema of the conjunctiva, and loss of eyelashes. Patients treated with PRT had a similar rate of acute toxicities, compared to patients treated with ERT. Cataracts were the most common long-term complication in eyes treated with EBRT. Other ocular complications noted are radiation retinopathy, glaucoma, neovascularization, vitreous hemorrhage, retinal detachment, strabismus, and less common toxicities [35–38].

The hypothalamus-pituitary axis is known to be affected in EBRT as it is exposed to radiation beams. Growth hormone deficiency and thyroid-stimulating hormone abnormality are noted in patients treated with EBRT. However, due to PRT physical properties that eliminate the radiation to midline structures, these adverse effects are noted to be less than in conventional radiation therapy. Therefore, endocrinopathies were almost limited in patients treated with PRT [38, 39].

Another adverse effect reported is craniofacial deformities where the facial and bony structures tend to be affected in EBRT. These include hypoplasia, hyperpigmentation, or soft tissue fibrosis. Long-term dentofacial anomalies have also been reported [36, 38, 40].

Risk of new cancers is a major concern in retinoblastoma patients treated with radiotherapy. The cumulative incidence of a second cancer at 50 years after diagnosis of retinoblastoma was 36% for hereditary retinoblastoma. Bone, nasal cavity, connective and soft tissue, and other neoplasms have been associated in retinoblastoma survivors who received EBRT. Osteosarcomas and soft tissue sarcomas are the most common tumors reported in irradiated patients reaching up to 76% of all cancer in ages younger than 25 years old. On the other hand, in unilateral retinoblastoma patients who did not receive radiation, sarcomas did not occur. In addition, the subsequent risk of cancer was noted to be higher in irradiated patients than nonirradiated whether the patients had hereditary or non-hereditary disease. Also, elevated doses of radiation were associated with increased risk of subsequent tumors. However, no subsequent cancers were noted among hereditary patients treated with chemotherapy. Furthermore, a comparison between photon and proton radiotherapy techniques was done and it showed that the 10-year cumulative incidence of malignancies was significantly higher in photon therapy compared to proton therapy. Therefore, patients treated with radiotherapy should have long follow-ups regardless of the modality used [32, 33, 41].

Lastly, the quality of life was observed, and no difference was noted between children and their parents regarding the quality-of-life outcomes compared to the general population [38].

5. Brachytherapy

Brachytherapy is a form of radiotherapy where a source of radiation is placed inside or next to the treatment area. In retinoblastoma the radioactive implant is placed on the sclera corresponding to the tumor base and fixed surgically to irradiate the tumor. Implantation technique requires excellent surgical skills and is applied under general sedation where the implant is fixed on the sclera and maintained for few days and removed with the patients remaining in the hospital during the entire treatment [42]. Iodine-125 and Ruthenium-106 are the most common radioactive agents to be used in intraocular lesions. Other agents can be used such as Ruthenium-106, Palladium-103, Strontium-90, Cobalt-60, and Iridium-192 [42, 43]. Like EBRT, the use of brachytherapy has been limited to progressive disease and to preserve the eye from enucleation. However, brachytherapy offers less spread of radiation, and its complications that can be associated with EBRT can be prevented where damage of normal tissue can be minimized which can lead to deformities and more importantly reduce the risk of radiation-induced second cancers [42, 44, 45]. Brachytherapy can be used as primary modality to treat retinoblastoma where the tumor is found solitary and located anterior to the equator as per the American Brachytherapy Society-Ophthalmic Oncology Task Force (ABS-OOTF) recommendations. As for secondary treatment where retinoblastoma failed to respond to other treatment modalities, it can be used irrespective of its location [43]. Brachytherapy is also an effective method that can be used post enucleation to prevent recurrence [46].

Plaque brachytherapy achieved tumor control in 83–89% of cases in some studies reaching up to 88% when used as a primary modality and appears to be the best choice in patients who failed laser photocoagulation, thermotherapy, cryotherapy, or chemoreduction, but it is less successful in patients who failed EBRT [45, 47, 48].

Reirradiation of local recurrence with brachytherapy can be considered as an option to salvage the eye from enucleation, and it may provide tumor control and eye preservation [48]. Complications related to radiation included radiation retinopathy, maculopathy, papillopathy, cataract, and glaucoma. Fortunately, no second cancers related to plaque brachytherapy were reported in the literature [45, 47–50].

Visual acuity in patients was found to be good in 64% and poor in 24–32% of non-enucleated eyes who were treated with plaque radiotherapy. The poor visual outcome was mainly associated with macular lesions, macular edema, vitreous hemorrhage, and phthisis bulbi. It appears that there is no significant difference whether brachytherapy was used as a primary or secondary modality in visual outcome [45, 47].

In many centers, Iodine-125 is used as the standard isotope for plaque brachytherapy. This is due to the physical properties like its half-life, low energy, adequate dose distribution, and ease of shielding [42, 43]. In a study, the use of Iodine-125 as salvage treatment in 84 recurrent lesions after chemoreduction is reported. It showed 95% control in those who failed chemoreduction and 100% control in patients who failed a combination of chemoreduction and EBRT. Complications were higher in patients who received EBRT and included papillopathy, vitreous hemorrhage, cataract, and neovascularization [50].

Ruthenium-106 has some advantages over Iodine-125 where it's lower in cost, has longer half-life, and is safer in terms of radioprotection. It has shown tumor control achievement up to 73%, and some studies achieved eye preservation in 89% of cases. Local recurrence with Ruthenium-106 is noted to reach 6.3%. Complications of Ruthenium-106 are generally similar to those found in other radiation modalities such as proliferative retinopathy which can lead to vitreous hemorrhage, radiation maculopathy radiation optic neuropathy, exudative retinal detachment, neovascularization, neovascular glaucoma, and cataracts. Previous treatment with EBRT was shown to be associated with increased risk of some complications such as optic neuropathy, retinal detachment, and cataracts. However, studies of efficacy of Ruthenium-106 in retinoblastoma compared to Iodine-125 are limited in the literature [51–54].

6. Focal therapy

Focal therapy in treatment of retinoblastoma is used either alone in small retinoblastomas (group A or B) (1, 2 laser) or after chemoreduction, usually after two or three cycles, or for small recurrent tumors or subretinal seeds [55–57].

7. Transpupillary thermotherapy (TTT)

Thermotherapy is based on increasing the tissue temperature from 45 to 60°C to induce a cytotoxic effect, through applying an 810-nm diode laser below the coagulative threshold to prevent retinal vessels from coagulation, and it can be used alone for small retinoblastomas that are 3 mm in diameter without vitreous or subretinal seeds [57, 58]. In a study of 91 tumors, 92% of the tumors that were 1.5 mm in diameter were controlled with thermotherapy alone [59]. Out of 188 treated by thermotherapy, complete regression of the tumor was achieved in (85%) 161 tumors, where the mean tumor size is 3.0 mm base and 2.0 mm thickness [60]. Complications of transpupillary thermotherapy include iris atrophy, cataracts, tumor seeding into the vitreous, retinal fibrosis, transition, and vascular occlusion.

8. Laser photocoagulation

Laser photocoagulation is aimed to diminish blood supply of tumor. This type of treatment is used for small (4 mm in diameter and 2 mm in thickness) and posterior tumors. Argon or diode laser or a xenon arc is used but not directly on tumor tissue; instead it is aimed to coagulate the blood vessels that supply the tumor.

Retinal detachment, retinal vascular occlusion, retinal traction, and preretinal fibrosis can be a complication of this type of treatment [61–63].

9. Cryotherapy

Cryotherapy induces rapid decrease (freeze) of tumor tissue, and this will cause damage to the tumor blood vessel endothelium and lead to vascular thrombosis, which results in tumor ischemia and infarction. It is used as primary treatment for small equatorial and peripheral retinal tumors (<3.5-mm base and <2-mm thickness). Treatment protocol is based on three applications for each session every 4–6 weeks until complete regression of the tumor. Complications of cryotherapy include retinal tears and detachment, proliferative vitreoretinopathy, and chorioretinal atrophy. Cryotherapy can be used 2–3 hours before chemotherapy administration, and that can increase the permeability of blood retinal barrier and increase the effect of chemotherapy [61, 63].

10. Chemotherapy

Chemotherapy is considered as one of the most important modalities used to treat retinoblastoma. It has been used as a main therapeutic modality achieving tumor control in up to 78% with the elimination of the need for enucleation as well as EBRT and its risk of developing second new cancers [64]. Chemotherapeutic agents can be delivered via four main routes which are intravenous chemotherapy, intra-arterial chemotherapy (IAC), intravitreal chemotherapy, and periocular chemotherapy. The most common chemotherapeutic agents used are vincristine, etoposide, and carboplatin. This (VEC) regimen is the most popular combination preferred by many experts, and this stems from its proven effect on neuronal tumors in the pediatric age group as well as its good penetration into the eye [65]. Melphalan is considered as the best and most effective agent in intra-arterial chemotherapy, and it is the most commonly used [66]. Tumor control, chemoreduction, and outcome differ from one modality and route of administration to another. Outcome also depends on the ICRB where chemotherapy can be successful in 100% in group A and it drops as low as 50% in groups D and E. Visual outcome can be maintained with a visual acuity of 6/60 or better in around two-thirds of patients [16, 67]. Adverse effects of chemotherapy observed are different from one modality to another. For instance, common side effects seen with systemic chemotherapy include transient pancytopenia, fever, and alopecia. Intra-arterial chemotherapy complications are attributed either to the procedure itself or to the chemotherapeutic agent. It can result in endovascular complications, allergy, and hematoma at the site of entry. IAC can also result in ocular vascular complications. Neutropenia is another important complication noted in IAC. Among the most frequent side effects of intravitreal chemotherapy are retinal pigment epithelium changes, iris depigmentation and atrophy, chorioretinal atrophy with vitreous hemorrhage, and retinal detachment. Fortunately, second primary malignancy risk in chemotherapy is almost eliminated compared to EBRT which has made chemotherapy more superior in treating retinoblastoma [68–75]. A more detailed information is mentioned in the chapter entitled Retinoblastoma Management: Advances in Chemotherapy.

Acknowledgements

The authors would like to thank King Khalid Eye Specialist Hospital for the photos provided, and Ophthalmology Department at King Abdulaziz University Hospital under King Saud University Institute for funding and supporting this chapter.

Conflict of interest

There is no financial interest to disclose.

Author details

Abdullah Almater[1*], Abdulrahman Alfaleh[1,2], Khalid Alshomar[1] and Saleh AlMesfer[3]

1 Department of Ophthalmology, College of Medicine, King Saud University, Riyadh, Saudi Arabia

2 Department of Ophthalmology, College of Medicine, Jouf University, Sakaka, Saudi Arabia

3 Division of Pediatric Ophthalmology, King Khaled Eye Specialist Hospital, Riyadh, Saudi Arabia

*Address all correspondence to: aim-93@hotmail.com

References

[1] Shields JA, Shields CL, Parsons HM. Differential diagnosis of retinoblastoma. Retina. 1991;**11**:232-243

[2] Shields JA, Augsburger JJ. Current approaches to the diagnosis and management of retinoblastoma. Survey of Ophthalmology. 1981;**25**:347-372

[3] Yoshizumi MO, Thomas JV, Smith TR. Glaucoma-inducing mechanisms in eyes with retinoblastoma. Archives of Ophthalmology. 1978;**96**:105-110

[4] Chintagumpala M, Chevez-Barrios P, Paysse EA, Plon SE, Hurwitz R. Retinoblastoma: Review of current management. The Oncologist. 2007;**12**:1237-1246

[5] Smith EV, Gragoudas ES, Kolodny NH, et al. Magnetic resonance imaging: An emerging technique for the diagnosis of ocular disorders. International Ophthalmology. 1990;**14**:119-124

[6] Brenner D, Elliston C, Hall E, et al. Estimated risks of radiation-induced fatal cancer from pediatric CT. AJR. American Journal of Roentgenology. 2001;**176**:289-296

[7] Kuker W, Ramaekers V. Persistent hyperplastic primary vitreous: MRI. Neuroradiology. 1999;**41**:520-522

[8] Kaste SC, Jenkins JJ 3rd, Meyer D, et al. Persistent hyperplastic primary vitreous of the eye: Imaging findings with pathologic correlation. AJR. American Journal of Roentgenology. 1994;**162**:437-440

[9] Chang MM, McLean IW, Merritt JC. Coats' disease: A study of 62 histologically confirmed cases. Journal of Pediatric Ophthalmology and Strabismus. 1984;**21**:163-168

[10] Morgan KS, McLean IW. Retinoblastoma and persistent hyperplastic vitreous occurring in the same patient. Ophthalmology. 1981;**88**:1087-1089

[11] Shields CL, Schoenberg E, Kocher K, et al. Lesions simulating retinoblastoma (pseudo retinoblastoma) in 604 cases: Results based on age at presentation. Ophthalmology. 2013;**120**:311-316

[12] Brierley JD, Gospodarowicz MK, Wittekind C, editors. Retinoblastoma. In: TNM Classification of Malignant Tumours. 8th ed. Oxford, UK: Wiley-Blackwell; 2017

[13] Mallipatna A, Gallie BL, Chévez-Barrios P, et al. Retinoblastoma. In: Amin MB, Edge SB, Greene FL, editors. AJCC Cancer Staging Manual. 8th ed. New York, NY: Springer; 2017. pp. 819-831

[14] Ellsworth RM. The practical management of retinoblastoma. Transactions of the American Ophthalmological Society. 1969; **67**:462-534

[15] Linn Murphree A. Intraocular retinoblastoma: The case for a new group classification. Ophthalmology Clinics of North America. 2005;**18**(1):41-53

[16] Shields CL, Mashayekhi A, Au AK, et al. The international classification of retinoblastoma predicts chemoreduction success. Ophthalmology. 2006;**113**(12):2276-2280

[17] Shields JA, Shields CL. Management and prognosis of retinoblastoma. In: Intraocular Tumors. A Text and Atlas. Philadelphia: WB Saunders; 1992. pp. 377-392

[18] Shields JA, Shields CL. Retinoblastoma. In: Shields JA, Shields CL, editors. Atlas of Intraocular Tumors.

Philadelphia: Lippincott Williams & Wilkins; 2008. pp. 293-365

[19] De Potter P, Shields CL, Shields JA, Singh AD. Use of the orbital hydroxyapatite implant in the pediatric population. Archives of Ophthalmology. 1994;**112**:208-212

[20] Shields CL, Uysal Y, Marr BP, et al. Experience with the polymer-coated hydroxyapatite implant following enucleation in 126 patients. Ophthalmology. 2007;**114**:367-373

[21] Mallipatna AC, Sutherland JE, Gallie BL, et al. Management and outcome of unilateral retinoblastoma. Journal of AAPOS. 2009;**13**:546-550

[22] Abramson DH. Treatment of retinoblastoma. In: Blodi FC, editor. Retinoblastoma. New York: Churchill Livingstone; 1985. pp. 3-93

[23] Zhao J, Dimaras H, Massey C, et al. Pre-enucleation chemotherapy for eyes severely affected by retinoblastoma masks risk of tumor extension and increases death from metastasis. Journal of Clinical Oncology. 2011;**29**:845-851

[24] Aerts I, Sastre-Garau X, Savignoni A, et al. Results of a multicenter prospective study on the postoperative treatment of unilateral retinoblastoma after primary enucleation. Journal of Clinical Oncology. 2013;**31**:1458-1463

[25] Shields CL, Shields JA. Retinoblastoma management: Advances in enucleation, intravenous chemoreduction, and intra-arterial chemotherapy. Current Opinion in Ophthalmology. 2010;**21**(3):203-212

[26] Uusitalo MS, Van Quill KR, Scott IU, et al. Evaluation of chemoprophylaxis in patients with unilateral retinoblastoma with high-risk features on histopathologic examination. Archives of Ophthalmology. 2001;**119**:41-48

[27] Honavar SG, Singh AD, Shields CL, et al. Postenucleation adjuvant therapy in high-risk retinoblastoma. Archives of Ophthalmology. 2002;**120**:923-931

[28] Eagle RC Jr. High-risk features and tumor differentiation in retinoblastoma: A retrospective histopathologic study. Archives of Pathology & Laboratory Medicine. 2009;**133**:12031209

[29] Shome D, Honavar SG, Raizada K, et al. Implant and prosthesis movement after enucleation: A randomized controlled trial. Ophthalmology. 2010;**117**:1638-1644

[30] Stannard C, Sauerwein W, Maree G, Lecuona K. Radiotherapy for ocular tumours. Eye (London, England). 2013;**27**(2):119-127

[31] Tian X, Liu K, Hou Y, Cheng J, Zhang J. The evolution of proton beam therapy: Current and future status. Molecular and Clinical Oncology. 2018;**8**(1):15-21

[32] Wong FL, Boice JD, Abramson DH, et al. Cancer incidence after retinoblastoma: Radiation dose and sarcoma risk. JAMA. 1997;**278**(15):1262-1267

[33] Kleinerman RA, Tucker MA, Tarone RE, et al. Risk of new cancers after radiotherapy in long-term survivors of retinoblastoma: An extended follow-up. Journal of Clinical Oncology. 2005;**23**(10):2272-2279

[34] Hall E. Radiobiology for the Radiologist. 5th ed. Philadelphia: Lippincott, Williams & Wilkins; 2000

[35] Agarwal A, Thaker NG, Tawk B, Allen PK, Grosshans DR, Herzog CE, et al. The evolution of radiation therapy for retinoblastoma: The MD Anderson cancer center experience. International Journal of Particle Therapy. 2016;**2**(4):490-498

[36] Choi SY, Kim MS, Yoo S, et al. Long term follow-up results of external beam radiotherapy as primary treatment for retinoblastoma. Journal of Korean Medical Science. 2010;**25**(4):546-551

[37] Mouw KW, Sethi RV, Yeap BY, et al. Proton radiation therapy for the treatment of retinoblastoma. International Journal of Radiation Oncology, Biology, Physics. 2014;**90**(4):863-869

[38] Mouw KW, Yeap BY, Caruso P, et al. Analysis of patient outcomes following proton radiation therapy for retinoblastoma. Advances in Radiation Oncology. 2017;**2**(1):44-52

[39] Pomarede R, Czernichow P, Zucker JM, et al. Incidence of anterior pituitary deficiency after radiotherapy at an early age: Study in retinoblastoma. Acta Paediatrica Scandinavica. 1984;**73**(1):115-119

[40] Khan S, Maheshwari S, Khan MT, Verma SK. Long term dento-facial effects of radiotherapy in a treated patient of retinoblastoma. Journal of Oral Biology and Craniofacial Research. 2014;**4**(3):214-217

[41] Sethi RV, Shih HA, Yeap BY, et al. Second nonocular tumors among survivors of retinoblastoma treated with contemporary photon and proton radiotherapy. Cancer. 2014;**120**(1):126-133

[42] Freire JE, De Potter P, Brady LW, Longton WA. Brachytherapy in primary ocular tumors. Seminars in Surgical Oncology. 1997;**13**(3):167-176

[43] Simpson ER, Gallie B, Laperrierre N, Beiki-Ardakani A, et al. The American Brachytherapy Society consensus guidelines for plaque brachytherapy of uveal melanoma and retinoblastoma. Brachytherapy. 2014;**13**(1):1-14

[44] Amendola BE, Lamm FR, Markoe AM, et al. Radiotherapy of retinoblastoma. A review of 63 children treated with different irradiation techniques. Cancer. 1990;**66**(1):21-26

[45] Shields CL, Shields JA, De Potter P, et al. Plaque radiotherapy in the management of retinoblastoma. Use as a primary and secondary treatment. Ophthalmology. 1993;**100**(2):216-224

[46] Stannard C, Sealy R, Hering E, et al. Postenucleation orbits in retinoblastoma: Treatment with 125I brachytherapy. International Journal of Radiation Oncology, Biology, Physics. 2002;**54**(5):1446-1454

[47] Shields CL, Shields JA, Minelli S, et al. Regression of retinoblastoma after plaque radiotherapy. American Journal of Ophthalmology. 1993;**115**(2):181-187

[48] Shields CL, Shields JA, Cater J, Othmane I, Singh AD, Micaily B. Plaque radiotherapy for retinoblastoma: Long-term tumor control and treatment complications in 208 tumors. Ophthalmology. 2001;**108**(11):2116-2121

[49] Gaspar de Souza Neves DF, Ferragut MA, Ferreira DV, et al. Reirradiation of the eye with plaque brachytherapy: A single institution experience report of eight consecutive patients submitted to retreatment after local relapse of malignant disease of the eye. Brachytherapy. 2014;**13**(3):281-284

[50] Shields CL, Mashayekhi A, Sun H, et al. Iodine 125 plaque radiotherapy as salvage treatment for retinoblastoma recurrence after chemoreduction in 84 tumors. Ophthalmology. 2006;**113**(11):2087-2092

[51] Abouzeid H, Moeckli R, Gaillard MC, et al. (106) Ruthenium brachytherapy for retinoblastoma. International Journal of Radiation Oncology, Biology, Physics. 2008;**71**(3):821-828

[52] Schueler AO, Flühs D, Anastassiou G, Jurklies C, Sauerwein W, Bornfeld N. Beta-ray brachytherapy of retinoblastoma: Feasibility of a new small-sized ruthenium-106 plaque. Ophthalmic Research. 2006;**38**(1):8-12

[53] Schueler AO, Flühs D, Anastassiou G, et al. Beta-ray brachytherapy with 106Ru plaques for retinoblastoma. International Journal of Radiation Oncology, Biology, Physics. 2006;**65**(4):1212-1221

[54] Summanen P, Immonen I, Kivelä T, Tommila P, Heikkonen J, Tarkkanen A. Radiation related complications after ruthenium plaque radiotherapy of uveal melanoma. The British Journal of Ophthalmology. 1996;**80**(8):732-739

[55] Shields CL, Honavar SG, Meadows AT, Shields JA, Demirci H, Naduvilath TJ. Chemoreduction for unilateral retinoblastoma. Archives of Ophthalmology. 2002;**120**:1653-1658

[56] Shields CL, Honavar SG, Meadows AT, et al. Chemoreduction plus focal therapy for retinoblastoma: Factors predictive of need for treatment with external beam radiotherapy or enucleation. American Journal of Ophthalmology. 2002;**133**:657-664

[57] Murphree AL, Villablanca JG, Deegan WF 3rd, et al. Chemotherapy plus local treatment in the management of intraocular retinoblastoma. Archives of Ophthalmology. 1996;**114**:1348-1356

[58] Murphree AL, Munier FL. Retinoblastoma. In: Ryan SJ, editor. Retina. 2nd ed. St Louis: Mosby-Year Book Inc.; 1994. pp. 605-606

[59] Abramson DH, Schefler AC. Transpupillary thermotherapy as initial treatment for small intraocular retinoblastoma: Technique and predictors of success. Ophthalmology. 2004;**111**:984-991

[60] Shields CL, Santos MC, Diniz W, et al. Thermotherapy for retinoblastoma. Archives of Ophthalmology. 1999;**117**:885-893

[61] Hamel P, Heon E, Gallie BL, Budning AS. Focal therapy in the management of retinoblastoma: When to start and when to stop. Journal of American Association for Pediatric Ophthalmology and Strabismus. 2000;**4**(6):334-337

[62] Shields JA, Shields CL. Current Management of Retinoblastoma. Mayo Clinic Proceedings. 1994;**69**(1):50-56

[63] Murthy R, Honavar SG, Naik MN, Reddy VA. Retinoblastoma. In: Dutta LC, editor. Modern Ophthalmology. New Delhi, India: Jaypee Brothers; 2004. pp. 849-859

[64] Shields CL, Mashayekhi A, Cater J, Shelil A, Meadows AT, Shields JA. Chemoreduction for retinoblastoma: Analysis of tumor control and risks for recurrence in 457 tumors. Transactions of the American Ophthalmological Society. 2004;**102**:35-44 discussion 44-5

[65] Shields CL, Meadows AT, Leahey AM, Shields JA. Continuing challenges in the management of retinoblastoma with chemotherapy. Retina. 2004;**24**(6):849-862

[66] Jabbour P, Chalouhi N, Tjoumakaris S, et al. Pearls and pitfalls of intraarterial chemotherapy for retinoblastoma. Journal of Neurosurgery. Pediatrics. 2012;**10**(3):175-181. DOI: 10.3171/2012.5.PEDS1277.

[67] Narang S, Mashayekhi A, Rudich D, Shields CL. Predictors of long-term visual outcome after chemoreduction for management of intraocular retinoblastoma. Clinical & Experimental Ophthalmology. 2012;**40**(7):736-742. DOI: 10.1111/j.1442-9071.2012.02757.x.

[68] Shields CL, Lally SE, Leahey AM, et al. Targeted retinoblastoma management: When to use intravenous, intra-arterial, periocular, and intravitreal chemotherapy. Current Opinion in Ophthalmology. 2014;**25**(5):374-385. DOI: 10.1097/ICU.0000000000000091.

[69] Zanaty M, Barros G, Chalouhi N, et al. Update on intra-arterial chemotherapy for retinoblastoma. Scientific World Journal. 2014;**2014**: 869604. DOI: 10.1155/2014/869604

[70] Wyse E, Handa JT, Friedman AD, Pearl MS. A review of the literature for intra-arterial chemotherapy used to treat retinoblastoma. Pediatric Radiology. 2016;**46**(9):1223-1233

[71] Munier FL, Gaillard MC, Balmer A, et al. Intravitreal chemotherapy for vitreous disease in retinoblastoma revisited: From prohibition to conditional indications. The British Journal of Ophthalmology. 2012;**96**(8):1078-1083

[72] Shields CL, Manjandavida FP, Arepalli S, Kaliki S, Lally SE, Shields JA. Intravitreal melphalan for persistent or recurrent retinoblastoma vitreous seeds: Preliminary results. JAMA Ophthalmology. 2014;**132**(3):319-325

[73] Smith SJ, Smith BD, Mohney BG. Ocular side effects following intravitreal injection therapy for retinoblastoma: A systematic review. The British Journal of Ophthalmology. 2014;**98**(3):292-297

[74] Habib LA, Francis JH, Fabius AW, Gobin PY, Dunkel IJ, Abramson DH. Second primary malignancies in retinoblastoma patients treated with intra-arterial chemotherapy: The first 10 years. The British Journal of Ophthalmology. 2018;**102**(2):272-275

[75] Turaka K, Shields CL, Meadows AT, Leahey A. Second malignant neoplasms following chemoreduction with carboplatin, etoposide, and vincristine in 245 patients with intraocular retinoblastoma. Pediatric Blood & Cancer. 2012;**59**(1):121-125

Chapter 6

Retinoblastoma Management: Advances in Chemotherapy

Amani Al Kofide and Eman Al-Sharif

Abstract

The treatment of children with retinoblastoma (RB) has evolved from primarily enucleation of the eye(s) to highly selective methods of chemotherapy administration and approach. Indulgent and comprehensive understanding of the multitude of factors including accurate classification and grading of disease, timing and response to therapy, when to consolidate with local methods of therapy, combination regimens to control systemic disease and prevent relapse while minimizing risk of secondary cancers are crucial factors in the management of children with retinoblastoma. Chemotherapy was introduced in the 1950s and has become an integral component in management of RB. Methods of administration range from systemic to locally directed therapy including; intravitreal, periocular and intra-arterial chemotherapy. This chapter is intended to discuss the evolution and current chemotherapeutic agents with various routes of administration. The indications, adverse occurrences, short- and long-term complications of both local and systemic treatments will be elucidated.

Keywords: chemotherapy, retinoblastoma, metastasis, intravenous, intra-arterial, intravitreal, periocular, vitreous seeds

1. Introduction

The treatment of retinoblastoma is challenging, as the governing objectives are preserving life, protecting from pineoblastoma, decreasing the lifetime incidence of secondary tumors and salvaging useful vision without exposing the patient to significant and serious side effects that may endanger the patient's survival and quality of life. The treatment of retinoblastoma evolved steadily during the past decades, and multiple modalities of treatment were introduced including chemotherapy. At one time, chemotherapy was used mainly to manage metastatic retinoblastoma, but later the interest of scientists and clinicians shifted to the use of this treatment strategy for non-metastatic retinoblastoma. As the interest of experts grew and the demand for better overall outcome increased, multiple interesting treatment strategies were developed and refined. Now, four main routes of administration of chemotherapy are present, and these are: intravenous chemotherapy (IVC), intra-arterial chemotherapy (IAC), intravitreal chemotherapy (IVitC) and periocular chemotherapy (POC).

Today, chemotherapy is regarded as one of the indispensable pillars of treatment of retinoblastoma. In fact, retinoblastoma is currently one of the most commonly curable childhood malignant tumors universally. In developed countries, the rates of expected survival exceed 95% whereas the rates in developing countries are lower due to the limited healthcare resources [1]. The different chemotherapy treatment strategies outlined above will be discussed thoroughly in the upcoming sections.

2. Intravenous chemotherapy for retinoblastoma

The era of chemotherapeutic treatment for retinoblastoma began in 1953 when Carl Kupfer reported the successful use of intravenous nitrogen mustard along with irradiation to treat a child with recurrent retinoblastoma [2]. Thereafter, the use of triethylene melamine, a chemotherapeutic alkylating agent, via different routes (oral, intramuscular, intravenous and intra-arterial) became more widespread between clinicians until the late 1960s given that it allowed the reduction of radiotherapy dose which was associated with multiple potential side effects [3–6]. In the following years, the use of systemic chemotherapy fluctuated until the early 1990s when the use of systemic chemotherapy was popularized and strongly advocated by the leading retinoblastoma treatment centers worldwide and the use of external beam radiation was restricted in favor of chemotherapy due to the considerable risk of secondary tumors in patients receiving radiotherapy.

The management of retinoblastoma should be carried out by an experienced team as these children need meticulous bilateral ocular examination, usually under anesthesia, in parallel with systemic evaluation by a pediatric oncologist with experience in ocular oncology and appropriate systemic imaging by magnetic resonance imaging (MRI) must be standardly performed to rule out metastasis. These steps are vital to accurately classify the disease in accordance with the more recent International Classification of Retinoblastoma (ICRB). This will direct the treatment to either systemic chemotherapy or local therapies (thermal, cryotherapy and chemotherapy) or a combination of both.

Understating the effect of systemic chemotherapy on the different forms of retinoblastoma (solid tumor, subretinal tumor and vitreous seeds) is essential as it helps in guiding the treatment. Moreover, the likely complications and systemic toxicities of IVC are important to be looked at carefully before commencement as this will help in individualizing the treatment in this vulnerable subset of patients so as to reduce systemic morbidities without jeopardizing the treatment success [7]. In this section, we will highlight the principal characteristics of this treatment modality.

2.1 Indications

The use of IVC varies slightly between different treatment centers worldwide; but generally speaking, the umbrella of IVC usage encompasses its use in patients with intraocular disease only and in patients with or at high risk of extraocular disease. When the disease is limited to the eyes, IVC aims at shrinking the size of the tumor to expedite cure and lessen the damage induced by consolidating local therapies to follow, especially when the tumor involves sensitive retinal areas such as the macula. This has been termed chemoreduction and it had been shown to achieve adequate tumor control (alone or along with focal consolidating therapies) and eliminate the need for enucleation or external beam radiation (EBR) in more than 75% of patients in a large series (n = 457, group A–D). The risk of recurrence in this series was 22% and these were usually detected in the first year after starting the treatment; yet; none occurred by 4 years of follow up [8, 9]. This is probably the most important concern arising with the use of chemoreduction; though continuous surveillance of these children partly helps in overcoming this shortcoming.

Moreover, one study suggested that the administration of chemoreduction might minimize the risk of pineoblastoma where none of the children (n = 147) receiving this therapy developed trilateral retinoblastoma [10].

IVC is used also as an adjuvant therapy after enucleation in patients with extraocular disease (metastasis) as well as patients with intraocular disease associated with high-risk histopathological features (e.g., optic nerve invasion beyond the lamina cribrosa and choroid invasion >3 mm) demonstrated on histopathological examination of the enucleated eye [11]. It is speculated that patients with high-risk features might presumably have micro-metastasis and administering systemic chemoprophylaxis helps in improving their prognosis. Evidence in the literature supports the use of prophylactic IVC in high-risk patients where it was shown that it is safe and effective in decreasing the risk of metastasis [12, 13].

Patients with extraocular disease receiving IVC can be divided into three categories: those with orbital and/or regional spread to the preauricular lymph nodes or optic nerve cut, those with central nervous system (CNS) dissemination and those with distant extracranial metastasis [14]. In patients presenting with orbital retinoblastoma, IVC is a valuable treatment. This holds true when it is predominantly administered in combination with other therapies (multimodal therapy: surgery, radiotherapy and chemotherapy) as its effect is usually inadequate when given alone [15]. Patients who have CNS involvement usually have a very poor prognosis with low survival rate. The usual approach to these patients consists of platinum-based IVC with agents having good CNS penetration along with focal CNS treatments such as radiotherapy. Some studies suggested using high doses of IVC followed by autologous hematopoietic progenitor cell rescue; yet, this technique is controversial [16]. Distant metastasis usually occurs to the bone and a small series (n = 14) on stage 4A patients showed promising results using intense induction chemotherapy followed by high dose consolidating chemotherapy and autologous hematopoietic progenitor cell rescue [17].

2.2 Chemotherapeutic protocol

Over the past decades, multiple chemotherapeutic agents were used, and multiple chemotherapy protocols were implemented, some of which are now outdated. In the meantime, the most commonly employed IVC therapy is the VEC protocol consisting of three main chemotherapeutic agents (Vincristine, Etoposide, Carboplatin) in standard doses based on the body weight. Higher doses may be used in patients with more advanced disease (bilateral group D or E) [7, 18]. This three-drug regimen is the most popular combination preferred by many experts and this stems from its proven effect on neuronal tumors in the pediatric age group as well as its good penetration into the eye [19]. The patient usually receives 6–9 cycles on a monthly basis and once the tumor shrinks in size, then focal consolidating treatments can follow [7].

2.3 Complications

Common side effects, which are usually observed with any systemic chemotherapy, include transient pancytopenia owing to bone marrow suppression, fever and alopecia. The occurrence of these side effects is usually limited to the treatment period. Although carboplatin, a platinum based agent, had been linked to ototoxicity and nephrotoxicity, these serious side effects are rare as they are dose-dependent [20, 21]. There was an underlying concern that etoposide may induce acute myelogenous leukemia especially with high multiple doses; yet, the results of several studies on this topic were reassuring [7, 22]. With regards to secondary tumors, it does not seem that IVC increases the risk ominously. A long term follow-up study demonstrated that the rate of secondary tumors in germline retinoblastoma patients treated with systemic chemotherapy was 4%, which is less than expected for this vulnerable subset of patients [23].

2.4 Outcomes and success rate

The introduction of systemic chemotherapy resulted in an improved eye salvage rate, not to mention the enhanced visual outcome. Chemoreduction success can be predicted in patients with retinoblastoma following the ICRB classification as following: 100% in group A, 93% in group B, 90% in group C and <50% in group D and E [24]. The success rate in the advanced stages can be augmented when combining IVC with other modalities of treatment such as IAC or IVitC. Long-term studies have shown that chemotherapy with or without adjunctive therapies maintains ambulatory vision of ≥6/60 in almost two-thirds of the patients, particularly those with multiple tumors and/or no foveolar tumors [25]. Furthermore, IVC seems to exert a protective effect against pineoblastoma as its occurrence is usually very low in patients receiving it [26].

The effect of systemic chemotherapy as a monotherapy appears to be satisfactory especially in patients with less advanced disease whereas in patients with advanced disease, its remedial action is complementary to the selective recent therapies. A recently published meta-analysis comparing IVC to the more selective IAC revealed that both methods are equivalent in terms of tumor recurrence and metastasis. IAC evidently had a higher total success rate and ocular sparing effect in group D patients compared to IVC [27]. Despite this, we believe that IVC will continue to be an integral part of the treatment regimen of retinoblastoma.

3. Intra-arterial chemotherapy for retinoblastoma

Intra-arterial chemotherapy (IAC), also known as ophthalmic artery chemosurgery (OAC), is an important treatment strategy for retinoblastoma that evolved rapidly and gained popularity worldwide. Today, this modality of treatment is being performed in many retinoblastoma treatment centers located in more than 45 countries across the globe [28]. This treatment modality was initially explored by Reese et al. [3] who directly injected the alkylating agent triethylene melamine (TEM) into the internal carotid artery; nevertheless, it was not until 2006 when Abramson and Gobin introduced the novel technique of super-selective ophthalmic artery catheterization via transfemoral artery approach which allowed immediate and effectual delivery of the administered agent (melphalan) into the diseased eye [29]. Thereafter, many oncology centers adopted this technique and started publishing their experience. In this section, we will be shedding the light on the important aspects and most recent results of IAC.

3.1 Indications

IAC opened the door to a new era in the treatment of retinoblastoma. The key exciting factor behind this local therapy is its ability to achieve adequate therapeutic intraocular concentrations of the delivered chemotherapeutic agents while minimizing the systemic toxicity induced by these infused drugs such as neutropenia and secondary tumors [30]. In view of this, IAC is utilized mainly in treating patients with intraocular disease without local or systemic spread. Previous studies on IAC have shown that it can be used successfully as a primary retinoblastoma treatment in naïve eyes (no previous therapy employed) or as a secondary treatment in eyes with recurrent or residual tumor after trying other treatment modalities such as systemic chemotherapy, external beam radiotherapy and others [29, 31–37]. Currently, the common indications for IAC in retinoblastoma patients include unilateral retinoblastoma that cannot be halted by local treatments alone (e.g., cryotherapy or laser photocoagulation) and advanced unilateral retinoblastoma (such as group D and E based on the ICRB) [30]. Several studies had previously reported the following advantages of using IAC in patients with group D retinoblastoma: better eye conservation rates and greater visual acuity compared to systemic chemotherapy, shorter treatment period and ability to repeat the therapy several times using multiple agents without endangering the patients' life and vision [28, 38]. It is also noteworthy to mention that IAC can save naïve eyes with advanced retinoblastoma from enucleation particularly when subretinal seeding is present (2 year ocular survival rate of 83%) [39]. Furthermore, IAC has a proven benefit even in patients presenting with advanced disease such as those having retinoblastoma-induced total or partial retinal detachment in which it can successfully achieve retinal re-attachment and thus help in preserving the eye and the life with the least possible side effects [40, 41].

Simultaneous IAC (tandem therapy) to both eyes consecutively is also a valuable and safe treatment method in patients with bilateral germline retinoblastoma whether used primarily or secondarily. This was demonstrated in two recent studies, which reported excellent globe salvage rates (ocular survival rate > 90%) even in patients with advanced disease. Despite that the safety profile of this simultaneous therapy was considerably high where no treatment-associated deaths occurred, these children were still at risk of secondary tumors such as pineoblastoma and this is probably attributed to their inherent genetic predisposition [42, 43].

3.2 IAC technique

The technique of IAC is carried out on patients who are generally anesthetized and is usually coordinated by a specialized and experienced oncology/radiology team. The common femoral artery on the ipsilateral treatment side is usually used to gain access to the internal carotid artery and then the ophthalmic artery (OA) is selectively catheterized under fluoroscopic guidance at its ostium (origin) while heparin is infused intravenously to prevent coagulation. Then, in order to verify the proper placement of the microcatheter, selective angiography is done by contrast infusion to delineate the vascular anatomy and ocular perfusion. Due to the variability of vascular territory anatomy and blood flow patterns, OA catheterization might fail and other routes are available, however, this is out of the scope of this chapter [34].

3.3 Chemotherapeutic agents

The most commonly used intra-arterial chemotherapeutic agent is melphalan, a potent alkylating agent. Melphalan is by far the strongest chemotherapeutic drug acting effectually against human retinoblastoma cells [44]. It is very safe when administered locally but very toxic when infused systemically due to the resultant severe myelosuppression [45]. In fact, it is currently considered an ideal agent due to its favorable safety profile, short half-life and ability to be used in combination with other agents to achieve greater tumor control when needed [34, 46]. Topotecan, a topoisomerase inhibitor, and carboplatin, an alkylating agent, are other agents that have been used alone or as a part of a multi-drug regimen in advanced cases that fail to respond to melphalan solitarily or in bilateral tandem therapy where the dose of melphalan is decreased to prevent systemic side effects [34].

3.4 Complications

Despite being a less invasive therapeutic intervention, IAC does carry some risk of complications, as it would be expected with any medical interventional procedure. Complications occurring after IAC are attributed either to the procedure itself or to the chemotherapeutic agent/agents or both. Complications developing from the procedure include endovascular complications occurring intraoperative, allergy to iodine and hematoma at the site of entry into the femoral artery. Systemic thromboembolic and hemorrhagic events (stroke, limb ischemia) are possible but their current reported overall occurrence is extremely scarce [30, 44]. Up to date, no procedure-related deaths had been reported. Theoretically speaking, since IAC targets chiefly the intraocular pathology, the risk of metastasis and secondary neoplasms remains unchanged or even might be increased, as this treatment is not intended to reach the systemic circulation in high concentrations. Experts studied the incidence of death due to retinoblastoma-associated metastasis in a cohort of patients treated over a 10-year period by IAC primarily or secondarily and found it to be negligible (<1%) [47]. Likewise, IAC was not associated with an increased rate of second primary malignancies (SPM) in a group of patients with germline retinoblastoma from one treatment center studied over a 10-year period (2006–2016) [48]. However, IAC is relatively a recent therapy; therefore, it is still premature to derive definite conclusions regarding the potential risk and studies with longer follow up periods are required.

Neutropenia is another important complication that should be recognized and managed early to prevent devastating complications. The local distribution of the drug has helped in limiting its occurrence to <15% [34, 49]. On the other hand, minor ocular side effects are common and these include: lids edema, blepharoptosis, temporary loss of the eyelashes and forehead hyperemia along the distribution of the supratrochlear artery [50]. Ocular vascular complications are among the universally feared local side effects. A recent review of 16 published studies reported that <2.5% had ophthalmic artery obstruction or occlusion, choroidal ischemia or atrophy and vasospasm [49]. These vascular events should be interpreted in the context of the clinical case given that these are usually sick eyes that might have received other local treatments that might contribute to the occurrence of such events. A recently published study looked at the incidence of vascular events and the variability of their occurrence when IAC is given primarily or secondarily and reported the following: overall vascular complications occur in 5% of eyes per infusion and no difference was observed when IAC is used as a primary or secondary therapy [51].

3.5 Outcomes and success rate

The body of evidence in the literature supporting the use of IAC has been growing persistently in the past decade. Impressively, the reported globe salvage rate is currently exceeding 90% without compromising patient's survival and the enucleation rate dropped to <10% [35, 52–54]. Even the rate of orbital recurrence was significantly higher in patients with advanced disease treated with enucleation compared to IAC and this further emphasizes the gainful outcome of IAC [55].

A major concern about the risk of recurrence after IAC treatment remains in spite of the success achieved by this treatment modality. A recent study from one of the pioneering centers utilizing IAC with 10 years experience reported that around 25% of eyes treated primarily with IAC might develop recurrence. The recurrence of the disease was observed to occur mainly in the first 12 months post-treatment; and therefore, close follow up with serial meticulous examination is recommended during this period. Surprisingly, the rate of recurrence was higher in eyes that received the drug through routes other than OA and in eyes with widely spaced treatments more than 4 weeks. The risk of recurrence was <10% by 2 years in eyes remaining disease free in the first year after IAC [52].

4. Intravitreal chemotherapy for retinoblastoma

Intravitreal chemotherapy (IVitC) is another well-established targeted therapy accounting for one of the important current treatment modalities for retinoblastoma manifesting vitreous seeds. Initial reports on IVitC date back to the 1960s where thiotepa was injected into the vitreous cavity of six eyes with retinoblastoma; yet the results were inconclusive due to the limited number of treated eyes [56]. Later, this method was revived by Kaneko and Suzuki who injected melphalan intravitreally in 41 eyes along with ocular hyperthermia to cure vitreous seeding with a notable resultant eye preservation rate of 51.3% [57]. The choice of melphalan was essentially based on in-vitro testing of 12 anti-neoplastic drugs, and melphalan proved to be the most effective against retinoblastoma cells [45]. Implementing this technique into current practice took several years and perhaps the major limiting factor was the fear of disseminating the cancer cells during injection with the risk of subsequent extraocular spread causing metastasis and death. This section will elaborate on the key qualities of this relatively new therapy.

4.1 Indications and contraindications for intravitreal chemotherapy

This local therapeutic technique is intended essentially to achieve the highest concentration of the delivered tumoricidal drug into the confined intraocular space adjacent to the tumor. IVitC is used as an adjunctive therapy to chemoreduction with systemic chemotherapy and IAC. The main indications for this treatment modality are the presence of active vitreous seeds that are either refractory to standard therapy or recurrent after pervious standard therapy [7]. The use of IVitC had also expanded lately to include patients with retinal and subretinal tumors where it had been shown to be successful in salvaging the globe of such patients [58].

On the other hands, contraindications preventing the execution of this procedure include tumors involving the ciliary body or extending up to the anterior segment, tumors filling the globe, retinal detachment and vitreous hemorrhage.

4.2 Intravitreal chemotherapy technique

Before proceeding with this treatment, it is critical to meticulously evaluate the pars plana clinically in all quadrants 360° looking for any tumor foci as that could pose a threat to safety if present due to the risk of spread while injecting. If visualization is difficult, then ultrasound biomicroscopy can be used to help in detection and affirmation [59].

The procedure is usually carried out in the operating room under sterile conditions while the child is under general anesthesia. The anti-cancerous drug, typically melphalan, is injected through the pars plana 3–3.5 mm from the limbus into the vitreous cavity using a small needle, preferably a 32 gauge-needle. This creates the smallest needle track that helps in reducing the risk of dissemination. The injection is rather done in a seed-free quadrant, 2 o'clock hours away from vitreous seeds to prevent the undesirable exteriorization of tumor cells. Furthermore, some experts advocate reducing the pressure inside the eye by paracentesis before inserting the needle to prevent the possible risk of microscopic tumor seeding. After injecting the drug and before exiting the tumor-harboring globe, triple freeze-thaw cryotherapy should be carried out concurrently at the injection site while withdrawing the needle. Then, uniform intraocular distribution of the drug is achieved by gentle shaking of the eye using forceps. Examination is usually performed at the end of the procedure to rule out possible acute complications such as retinal detachment and bleeding. The ocular surface is then washed with balanced salt solution to remove any remnant chemotherapeutic agent that could be toxic. The child is usually discharged in the same day and the family is instructed to avoid touching the eye [59]. The procedure may vary minimally between different specialized treatment centers.

4.3 Chemotherapeutic agents

Melphalan hydrochloride is the principal drug injected into the vitreous cavity in retinoblastoma patients. It is a cytotoxic nitrogen mustard derivative that inhibits the synthesis of DNA and RNA together [59]. Its effective dosage range was studied and set at 20–30 μg per injection as low doses (8 μg) were not adequate to control and eradicate the disease while high doses (50 μg) controlled the disease but resulted in local toxicity (cataract, posterior segment hemorrhage, hypotony and phthisis bulbi) [60]. The number of injections is governed by the response. In general, Shields et al. proposed giving a total of six injections weekly or every 2 weeks [7].

Topotecan, a topoisomerase-1 inhibitor, is another potent intravitreal agent that had been employed in the treatment of retinoblastoma with vitreous seeds. Experimental animal studies showed that topotecan produce high and stable levels in the vitreous [61]. One of the distinguishable advantages of topotecan is its ability to attain a vitreous-to-plasma concentration five times more than melphalan [62]. Previous studies have shown that it is an effective anti-tumor drug with good safety profile and low ocular toxicity [63]. It had been used intravitreally in combination with melphalan in humans with encouraging results where this multi-agent regimen managed to achieve notable vitreous seeds regression with fewer injections [64]. Topotecan can also be used effectively in patients with recurrent or resistant viable vitreous seeds according to a recent study on 17 eyes which demonstrated control of these seeds in all treated eyes (100%) in the absence of ocular or systemic side effects and with a lower number of injections [65].

4.4 Complications

Extraocular tumor dissemination through the needle track with subsequent metastasis was perhaps the most feared serious event limiting the use of this treatment modality in the past. However, a meta-analysis examining published studies on this matter revealed that the risk of systemic spread is very low (two cases out of 1304 injections, proportion of extraocular spread secondary to injections was 0.007) especially when the appropriate safety enhancing injection techniques are applied. Therefore, IVitC can be utilized unreservedly whenever needed after proper patient selection [66].

Ocular side effects are generally uncommon in patients receiving IVitC. The major factor influencing the risk of complications and local ocular toxicity is the dose of administered medication where toxicity is more likely with melphalan doses higher than 30 μg [67]. Among the most frequent side effects is retinal pigment epithelium changes (salt and pepper retinopathy), which is believed to represent a form of chemical burn to the retinal at the area where the drug is concentrated the most [68, 69]. Retinal function decline due to toxicity, usually highlighted on electroretinography (ERG), is a possible complication of melphalan although the results are conflicting in the literature where one study showed no effect on ERG (dose:

20–30 μg) while another reported non-progressive decreased ERG amplitudes of approximately 5 μV (equivalent to 5% retinal response) with every 30 μg melphalan injection [70–72]. ERG can actually be a useful tool to monitor these patients for cumulative retinal toxicity.

Other major ocular complications that were highlighted in a systematic review with a total of 1287 intravitreal injections given to 306 eyes include: iris depigmentation and atrophy, chorioretinal atrophy with vitreous hemorrhage and retinal detachment [67]. Fortunately, there are no reports of endophthalmitis after IVitC; nonetheless, all protective measures should be taken to prevent this possible devastating complication.

With regards to serious systemic side effects, namely significant neutropenia of grade 3 and 4, these were not observed when analyzing 46 blood samples withdrawn from patients receiving IVitC (despite some patients received concurrent IAC) [71]. Again, this accentuates the benefit of local therapies in these young children.

4.5 Outcomes and success rate

Treating retinoblastoma with vitreous seeding can be really challenging due to the avascular nature of the vitreous; and therefore, drug delivery through systemic routes may not be sufficient sometimes. Besides this, it tends to be resistant to external radiation and systemic chemotherapy [68, 73]. In the past two decades, a quantum leap forward in the management of advanced retinoblastoma was reached with the help of IVitC. The reported vitreous seeding control rates of IVitC (melphalan with or without topotecan) ranges between 60 and 100% [60, 68, 71, 72, 74]. Additionally, the attained globe salvage rates are also impressive reaching up to 100% as reported in one study on 11 eyes receiving a total of 55 intravitreal melphalan injections [69].

5. Periocular chemotherapy for retinoblastoma

Periocular chemotherapy (POC) administration was designed to allow delivery of a higher concentration of the tumoricidal drugs locally. This route was firstly tested in retinoblastoma animal models using carboplatin and it had been shown that this route produces vitreous concentrations 8–10 folds more than the intravenous route [75, 76]. These preclinical results led to the conduction of a trial in which children with retinoblastoma were treated using subconjunctival carboplatin and the results were promising [77]. Thereafter, POC grew in popularity and it was consequently incorporated into the multimodal treatment algorithm of retinoblastoma. Currently, it is a part of the prospective multicenter Children's Oncology Group trials for retinoblastoma. In this section, POC will be tackled comprehensively.

5.1 Indications for periocular chemotherapy

POC is used predominantly as an adjunctive therapy to systemic chemotherapy as presently there is no evidence promoting it as a stand-alone therapy [78]. It is indicated principally in patients with recurrent localized tumor and in advanced disease (group D and E) where chemotherapy can be desirably infused in higher concentrations without exposing the patient to increased systemic toxicity [7]. It can also be utilized in patients who are not fit to receive systemic chemotherapy as well as patients with recurrent or persistent viable non-calcified vitreous seeds [78].

5.2 Chemotherapeutic agents

The common chemotherapeutic agents that are mostly used are carboplatin and topotecan. Experimental work showed that carboplatin peaks in the vitreous after 30 min of periocular injection and lasts for hours. Its concentration in the vitreous is approximately seven times more than that achieved by intravenous chemotherapy [76]. Several periocular drug administrative devices were explored and these include: plain liquid, Lincoff balloon, fibrin sealant, nanoparticles and iontophoresis [76, 79–81].

5.3 Complications

This treatment modality fortunately has no systemic side effects. Ocular complications do occur, and these mostly affect the periorbital tissue possibly owing to local toxicity. The most common observed side effects are lid edema, lid erythema, periorbital pseudocellulitis, ptosis, orbital fat atrophy, optic nerve atrophy and muscle fibrosis causing ocular motility changes [7, 77, 78, 82, 83]. Concerns were raised regarding the toxic effect on the extraocular muscles; yet, a study examining the effect of sub-tenon topotecan on the extraocular muscles of 10 eyes concluded that it had no toxic effect on the muscles and it is a safe and effective alternative [84].

5.4 Outcomes and success rate

Although the number of studies on POC is limited overall, it had been shown that POC is principally effective when combined with other modalities of anti-neoplastic therapies. One long-term follow up study demonstrated that 39% (n = 33 eyes) of the enrolled eyes were saved when treated with POC in addition to other concurrent treatment modalities. The same report indicated that two eyes treated by POC as monotherapy were cured and remained disease free on follow up [82].

6. Conclusions

In the last two decades, significant new approaches have been employed in the treatment of retinoblastoma which is a curable disease when diagnosed early. Modalities to avoid enucleation and minimize the short and long term effects of exposure to systemic chemotherapy and radiation therapy continue to evolve and now set the platform in the treatment of retinoblastoma. Despite new techniques such as selective intra-arterial and intravitreal chemotherapy, it is paramount to individualize therapy according to multiple factors including patient age, tumor location, stage of disease, size, and extension, along with realistic visual expectations. Personalized medicine will be able to tailor therapy with the best response and safety in children with retinoblastoma.

Acknowledgements

We would like to thank the College of Medicine Research Center, Deanship of Scientific Research, and Ophthalmology Department at King AbdulAziz University Hospital under King Saud University, Riyadh, Saudi Arabia for funding and supporting this chapter.

Conflict of interest

The authors have no conflict of interest to disclose.

Author details

Amani Al Kofide[1]* and Eman Al-Sharif[2]

1 Department of Pediatric Hematology/Oncology, King Faisal Specialist Hospital and Research Centre (Gen. Org.), Riyadh, Saudi Arabia

2 Department of Ophthalmology, College of Medicine, King Saud University, Riyadh, Saudi Arabia

*Address all correspondence to: kofide@kfshrc.edu.sa

References

[1] Shields CL, Shields JA. Diagnosis and management of retinoblastoma. Cancer Control. 2004;**11**:317-327

[2] Kupfer C. Retinoblastoma treated with intravenous nitrogen mustard. American Journal of Ophthalmology. 1953;**36**(12):1721-1723

[3] Reese AB, Hyman GA, Merriam GR Jr, Forrest AW, Kligerman MM. Treatment of retinoblastoma by radiation and triethylenemelamine. A.M.A. Archives of Ophthalmology. 1954;**53**(4):505-513

[4] Reese AB, Hyman GA, Tapley NA, Forrest AQ. The treatment of retinoblastoma by X-ray and triethylene melamine. A.M.A. Archives of Ophthalmology. 1958;**60**(5):897-906

[5] Krementz ET, Schlosser JV, Rumage JP, Herring L. Retinoblastoma: Behavior and treatment with fractional irradiation and intra-arterial triethylenemelamine. Annals of the New York Academy of Sciences. 1964;**114**(2):963-975

[6] Hyman GA, Ellsworth RM, Feind CR, Tretter P. Combination therapy in retinoblastoma: A 15-year summary of methods and results. Archives of Ophthalmology. 1968;**80**(6):744-746. DOI: 10.1001/archopht.1968.00980050746012

[7] Shields CL, Lally SE, Leahey AM, et al. Targeted retinoblastoma management: When to use intravenous, intra-arterial, periocular, and intravitreal chemotherapy. Current Opinion in Ophthalmology. 2014;**25**(5):374-385. DOI: 10.1097/ICU.0000000000000091

[8] Shields CL, De Potter P, Himelstein B, Shields JA, Meadows AT, Maris JM. Chemoreduction in the initial management of intraocular retinoblastoma. Archives of Ophthalmology. 1996;**114**:1330-1338

[9] Shields CL, Mashayekhi A, Cater J, Shelil A, Meadows AT, Shields JA. Chemoreduction for retinoblastoma: Analysis of tumor control and risks for recurrence in 457 tumors. Transactions of the American Ophthalmological Society. 2004;**102**:35-44. discussion 44-45

[10] Shields CL, Meadows AT, Shields JA, Carvalho C, Smith AF. Chemoreduction for retinoblastoma may prevent intracranial neuroblastic malignancy (trilateral retinoblastoma). Archives of Ophthalmology. 2001;**119**(9):1269-1272. DOI: 10.1001/archopht.119.9.1269

[11] Eagle RC Jr. High-risk features and tumor differentiation in retinoblastoma: A retrospective histopathologic study. Archives of Pathology & Laboratory Medicine. 2009;**133**(8):1203-1209. DOI: 10.1043/1543-2165-133.8.1203

[12] Honavar SG, Singh AD, Shields CL, et al. Postenucleation adjuvant therapy in high-risk retinoblastoma. Archives of Ophthalmology. 2002;**120**(7):923-931

[13] Kaliki S, Shields CL, Rojanaporn D, et al. High-risk retinoblastoma based on international classification of retinoblastoma: Analysis of 519 enucleated eyes. Ophthalmology. 2013;**120**(5):997-1003. DOI: 10.1016/j.ophtha.2012.10.044

[14] Rodriguez-Galindo C, Orbach DB, VanderVeen D. Retinoblastoma. Pediatric Clinics of North America. 2015;**62**(1):201-223. DOI: 10.1016/j.pcl.2014.09.014

[15] Honavar SG, Manjandavida FP, Reddy VAP. Orbital retinoblastoma: An update. Indian Journal of Ophthalmology. 2017;**65**(6):435-442

[16] Namouni F, Doz F, Tanguy ML, et al. High-dose chemotherapy with carboplatin, etoposide and cyclophosphamide followed by a haematopoietic stem cell rescue in patients with high-risk retinoblastoma: A SFOP and SFGM study. European Journal of Cancer. 1997;**33**(14):2368-2375

[17] Dunkel IJ, Khakoo Y, Kernan NA, et al. Intensive multimodality therapy for patients with stage 4a metastatic retinoblastoma. Pediatric Blood & Cancer. 2010;**55**:55-59

[18] Shields CL, Fulco EM, Arias JD, et al. Retinoblastoma frontiers with intravenous, intra-arterial, periocular, and intravitreal chemotherapy. Eye (London, England). 2013;**27**(2):253-264. DOI: 10.1038/eye.2012.175

[19] Shields CL, Meadows AT, Leahey AM, Shields JA. Continuing challenges in the management of retinoblastoma with chemotherapy. Retina. 2004;**24**(6):849-862

[20] Lambert MP, Shields C, Meadows AT. A retrospective review of hearing in children with retinoblastoma treated with carboplatin-based chemotherapy. Pediatric Blood & Cancer. 2008;**50**(2):223-226

[21] Leahey A. A cautionary tale: Dosing chemotherapy in infants with retinoblastoma. Journal of Clinical Oncology. 2012;**30**(10):1023-1024. DOI: 10.1200/JCO.2011.39.4254

[22] Gombos DS, Hungerford J, Abramson DH, et al. Secondary acute myelogenous leukemia in patients with retinoblastoma: Is chemotherapy a factor? Ophthalmology. 2007;**114**:1378-1383

[23] Turaka K, Shields CL, Meadows AT, Leahey A. Second malignant neoplasms following chemoreduction with carboplatin, etoposide, and vincristine in 245 patients with intraocular retinoblastoma. Pediatric Blood & Cancer. 2012;**59**(1):121-125. DOI: 10.1002/pbc.23278

[24] Shields CL, Mashayekhi A, Au AK, et al. The international classification of retinoblastoma predicts chemoreduction success. Ophthalmology. 2006;**113**(12): 2276-2280

[25] Narang S, Mashayekhi A, Rudich D, Shields CL. Predictors of long-term visual outcome after chemoreduction for management of intraocular retinoblastoma. Clinical & Experimental Ophthalmology. 2012;**40**(7):736-742. DOI: 10.1111/j.1442-9071.2012.02757.x

[26] Ramasubramanian A, Kytasty C, Meadows AT, Shields JA, Leahey A, Shields CL. Incidence of pineal gland cyst and pineoblastoma in children with retinoblastoma during the chemoreduction era. American Journal of Ophthalmology. 2013;**156**(4):825-829. DOI: 10.1016/j.ajo.2013.05.023

[27] Chen Q, Zhang B, Dong Y, et al. Comparison between intravenous chemotherapy and intra-arterial chemotherapy for retinoblastoma: A meta-analysis. BMC Cancer. 2018;**18**(1):486. DOI: 10.1186/s12885-018-4406-6

[28] Abramson DH, Daniels AB, Marr BP, et al. Intra-arterial chemotherapy (ophthalmic artery chemosurgery) for group D retinoblastoma. PLoS One. 2016;**11**(1):e0146582. DOI: 10.1371/journal.pone.0146582

[29] Abramson DH, Dunkel IJ, Brodie SE, Kim JW, Gobin YP. A phase I/II study of direct intraarterial (ophthalmic artery) chemotherapy with melphalan for intraocular retinoblastoma initial results. Ophthalmology.

2008;**115**(8):1398-1404. 1404.e1. DOI: 10.1016/j.ophtha.2007.12.014

[30] Zanaty M, Barros G, Chalouhi N, et al. Update on intra-arterial chemotherapy for retinoblastoma. Scientific World Journal. 2014;**2014**:869604. DOI: 10.1155/2014/869604

[31] Abramson DH, Dunkel IJ, Brodie SE, Marr B, Gobin YP. Superselective ophthalmic artery chemotherapy as primary treatment for retinoblastoma (chemosurgery). Ophthalmology. 2010;**117**(8):1623-1629. DOI: 10.1016/j.ophtha.2009.12.030

[32] Aziz HA, Boutrid H, Murray TG, et al. Supraselective injection of intraarterial melphalan as the primary treatment for late presentation unilateral multifocal stage Vb retinoblastoma. Retina. 2010;**30**(4 Suppl):S63-S65. DOI: 10.1097/IAE.0b013e3181cbda0f

[33] Say EA, Iyer PG, Hasanreisoglu M, et al. Secondary and tertiary intra-arterial chemotherapy for massive persistent or recurrent subretinal retinoblastoma seeds following previous chemotherapy exposure: Long-term tumor control and globe salvage in 30 eyes. Journal of AAPOS. 2016;**20**(4):337-342. DOI: 10.1016/j.jaapos.2016.05.009

[34] Gobin YP, Dunkel IJ, Marr BP, Brodie SE, Abramson DH. Intra-arterial chemotherapy for the management of retinoblastoma: Four-year experience. Archives of Ophthalmology. 2011;**129**(6):732-737. DOI: 10.1001/archophthalmol.2011.5

[35] Shields CL, Manjandavida FP, Lally SE, et al. Intra-arterial chemotherapy for retinoblastoma in 70 eyes: Outcomes based on the international classification of retinoblastoma. Ophthalmology. 2014;**121**(7):1453-1460. DOI: 10.1016/j.ophtha.2014.01.026

[36] Shields CL, Say EA, Pointdujour-Lim R, Cao C, Jabbour PM, Shields JA. Rescue intra-arterial chemotherapy following retinoblastoma recurrence after initial intra-arterial chemotherapy. Journal Français d'Ophtalmologie. 2015;**38**(6):542-549. DOI: 10.1016/j.jfo.2015.03.004

[37] Shields CL, Kaliki S, Shah SU, et al. Minimal exposure (one or two cycles) of intra-arterial chemotherapy in the management of retinoblastoma. Ophthalmology. 2012;**119**(1):188-192. DOI: 10.1016/j.ophtha.2011.06.036

[38] Munier FL, Mosimann P, Puccinelli F, et al. First-line intra-arterial versus intravenous chemotherapy in unilateral sporadic group D retinoblastoma: Evidence of better visual outcomes, ocular survival and shorter time to success with intra-arterial delivery from retrospective review of 20 years of treatment. The British Journal of Ophthalmology. 2017;**101**(8):1086-1093. DOI: 10.1136/bjophthalmol-2016-309298

[39] Abramson DH, Marr BP, Dunkel IJ, et al. Intra-arterial chemotherapy for retinoblastoma in eyes with vitreous and/or subretinal seeding: 2-year results. The British Journal of Ophthalmology. 2012;**96**:499-502

[40] Rowlands MA, Mondesire-Crump I, Levin A, et al. Total retinal detachments due to retinoblastoma: Outcomes following intra-arterial chemotherapy/ophthalmic artery chemosurgery. PLoS One. 2018;**13**(4):e0195395. DOI: 10.1371/journal.pone.0195395

[41] Shields CL, Kaliki S, Shah SU, Bianciotto CG, Jabbour P, Shields JA. Effect of intraarterial chemotherapy on retinoblastoma-induced retinal detachment. Retina. 2012;**32**(4):799-804. DOI: 10.1097/IAE.0b013e31823d8e1e

[42] Francis JH, Roosipu N, Levin AM, et al. Current treatment of bilateral retinoblastoma: The impact of intraarterial and intravitreous chemotherapy. Neoplasia. 2018;**20**(8):757-763. DOI: 10.1016/j.neo.2018.05.007

[43] Abramson DH, Marr BP, Francis JH, et al. Simultaneous bilateral ophthalmic artery chemosurgery for bilateral retinoblastoma (tandem therapy). PLoS One. 2016;**11**(6):e0156806

[44] Jabbour P, Chalouhi N, Tjoumakaris S, et al. Pearls and pitfalls of intraarterial chemotherapy for retinoblastoma. Journal of Neurosurgery. Pediatrics. 2012;**10**(3):175-181. DOI: 10.3171/2012.5.PEDS1277

[45] Inomata M, Kaneko A. Chemosensitivity profiles of primary and cultured human retinoblastoma cells in a human tumor clonogenic assay. Japanese Journal of Cancer Research. 1987;**78**(8):858-868

[46] Shields CL, Bianciotto CG, Jabbour P, et al. Intra-arterial chemotherapy for retinoblastoma: Report No. 1, control of retinal tumors, subretinal seeds, and vitreous seeds. Archives of Ophthalmology. 2011;**129**(11):1399-1406. DOI: 10.1001/archophthalmol.2011.150

[47] Abramson DH, Shields CL, Jabbour P, et al. Metastatic deaths in retinoblastoma patients treated with intraarterial chemotherapy (ophthalmic artery chemosurgery) worldwide. International Journal of Retina and Vitreous. 2017;**3**:40. DOI: 10.1186/s40942-017-0093-8

[48] Habib LA, Francis JH, Fabius AW, Gobin PY, Dunkel IJ, Abramson DH. Second primary malignancies in retinoblastoma patients treated with intra-arterial chemotherapy: The first 10 years. The British Journal of Ophthalmology. 2018;**102**(2):272-275. DOI: 10.1136/bjophthalmol-2017-310328

[49] Wyse E, Handa JT, Friedman AD, Pearl MS. A review of the literature for intra-arterial chemotherapy used to treat retinoblastoma. Pediatric Radiology. 2016;**46**(9):1223-1233. DOI: 10.1007/s00247-016-3554-6

[50] Abramson DH. Chemosurgery for retinoblastoma: What we know after 5 years. Archives of Ophthalmology. 2011;**129**(11):1492-1494. DOI: 10.1001/archophthalmol.2011.354

[51] Ancona-Lezama D, Dalvin LA, Lucio-Alvarez JA, Jabbour P, Shields CL. Ophthalmic vascular events after intra-arterial chemotherapy for retinoblastoma: Real-world comparison between primary and secondary treatments. Retina. Sep 7, 2018. DOI: 10.1097/IAE.0000000000002315 [Online ahead of print]

[52] Francis JH, Levin AM, Zabor EC, Gobin YP, Abramson DH. Ten-year experience with ophthalmic artery chemosurgery: Ocular and recurrence-free survival. PLoS One. 2018;**13**(5):e0197081. DOI: 10.1371/journal.pone.0197081

[53] Abramson DH, Shields CL, Munier FL, Chantada GL. Treatment of retinoblastoma in 2015: Agreement and disagreement. JAMA Ophthalmology. 2015;**133**(11):1341-1347

[54] Abramson DH, Fabius AW, Issa R, et al. Advanced unilateral retinoblastoma: The impact of ophthalmic artery chemosurgery on enucleation rate and patient survival at MSKCC. PLoS One. 2015;**10**(12):e0145436. DOI: 10.1371/journal.pone.0145436

[55] Yannuzzi NA, Francis JH, Marr BP, et al. Enucleation vs ophthalmic artery

chemosurgery for advanced intraocular retinoblastoma: A retrospective analysis. JAMA Ophthalmology. 2015;**133**(9):1062-1066

[56] Ericson LA, Rosengren BH. Present therapeutic resources in retinoblastoma. Acta Ophthalmologica. 1961;**39**:569-576

[57] Kaneko A, Suzuki S. Eye-preservation treatment of retinoblastoma with vitreous seeding. Japanese Journal of Clinical Oncology. 2003;**33**:601-607

[58] Abramson DH, Ji X, Francis JH, Catalanotti F, Brodie SE, Habib L. Intravitreal chemotherapy in retinoblastoma: Expanded use beyond intravitreal seeds. The British Journal of Ophthalmology. 2019;**103**(4):488-493. DOI: 10.1136/bjophthalmol-2018-312037

[59] Manjandavida FP, Shields CL. The role of intravitreal chemotherapy for retinoblastoma. Indian Journal of Ophthalmology. 2015;**63**(2):141-145

[60] Ghassemi F, Shields CL. Intravitreal melphalan for refractory or recurrent vitreous seeding from retinoblastoma. Archives of Ophthalmology. 2012;**130**(10):1268-1271

[61] Buitrago E, Del Sole MJ, Torbidoni A, et al. Ocular and systemic toxicity of intravitreal topotecan in rabbits for potential treatment of retinoblastoma. Experimental Eye Research. 2013;**108**:103-109. DOI: 10.1016/j.exer.2013.01.002

[62] Nemeth KM, Federico S, Carcaboso AM, et al. Subconjunctival carboplatin and systemic topotecan treatment in preclinical models of retinoblastoma. Cancer. 2010;**117**(2):421-434

[63] Schaiquevich P, Carcaboso AM, Buitrago E, et al. Ocular pharmacology of topotecan and its activity in retinoblastoma. Retina. 2014;**34**(9):1719-1727. DOI: 10.1097/IAE.0000000000000253

[64] Ghassemi F, Shields CL, Ghadimi H, Khodabandeh A, Roohipoor R. Combined intravitreal melphalan and topotecan for refractory or recurrent vitreous seeding from retinoblastoma. JAMA Ophthalmology. 2014;**132**(8):936-941. DOI: 10.1001/jamaophthalmol.2014.414

[65] Rao R, Honavar SG, Sharma V, Reddy VAP. Intravitreal topotecan in the management of refractory and recurrent vitreous seeds in retinoblastoma. The British Journal of Ophthalmology. 2018;**102**(4):490-495. DOI: 10.1136/bjophthalmol-2017-310641

[66] Smith SJ, Smith BD. Evaluating the risk of extraocular tumour spread following intravitreal injection therapy for retinoblastoma: A systematic review. The British Journal of Ophthalmology. 2013;**97**(10):1231-1236. DOI: 10.1136/bjophthalmol-2013-303188

[67] Smith SJ, Smith BD, Mohney BG. Ocular side effects following intravitreal injection therapy for retinoblastoma: A systematic review. The British Journal of Ophthalmology. 2014;**98**(3):292-297. DOI: 10.1136/bjophthalmol-2013-303885

[68] Munier FL, Gaillard MC, Balmer A, et al. Intravitreal chemotherapy for vitreous disease in retinoblastoma revisited: From prohibition to conditional indications. The British Journal of Ophthalmology. 2012;**96**(8):1078-1083

[69] Shields CL, Manjandavida FP, Arepalli S, Kaliki S, Lally SE, Shields JA. Intravitreal melphalan for persistent or recurrent retinoblastoma vitreous seeds: Preliminary results. JAMA Ophthalmology. 2014;**132**(3):319-325

[70] Brodie SE, Munier FL, Francis JH, Marr B, Gobin YP, Abramson DH.

Persistence of retinal function after intravitreal melphalan injection for retinoblastoma. Documenta Ophthalmologica. 2013;**126**(1):79-84

[71] Francis JH, Schaiquevich P, Buitrago E, et al. Local and systemic toxicity of intravitreal melphalan for vitreous seeding in retinoblastoma: A preclinical and clinical study. Ophthalmology. 2014;**121**(9):1810-1817

[72] Francis JH, Brodie SE, Marr B, Zabor EC, Mondesire-Crump I, Abramson DH. Efficacy and toxicity of Intravitreous chemotherapy for retinoblastoma: Four-year experience. Ophthalmology. 2017;**124**(4):488-495. DOI: 10.1016/j.ophtha.2016.12.015

[73] Francis JH, Habib LA, Abramson DH. Vitreous disease in retinoblastoma: Clinical findings and treatment. Advances in ophthalmology and optometry. 2017;**2**(1):177-195

[74] Suzuki S, Aihara Y, Fujiwara M, Sano S, Kaneko A. Intravitreal injection of melphalan for intraocular retinoblastoma. Japanese Journal of Ophthalmology. 2015;**59**(3):164-172. DOI: 10.1007/s10384-015-0378-0

[75] Harbour JW, Murray TG, Hamasaki D, et al. Local carboplatin therapy in transgenic murine retinoblastoma. Investigative Ophthalmology & Visual Science. 1996;**37**:1892-1898

[76] Mendelsohn ME, Abramson DH, Madden T, Tong W, Tran HT, Dunkel IJ. Intraocular concentrations of chemotherapeutic agents after systemic or local administration. Archives of Ophthalmology. 1998;**116**(9):1209-1212

[77] Abramosn DH, Frank CM, Dunkel IJ. A phase I/II study of subconjunctival carboplatin for intraocular retinoblastoma. Ophthalmology. 1999;**106**(10):1947-1950

[78] Kaliki S, Shields CL. Retinoblastoma: Achieving new standards with methods of chemotherapy. Indian Journal of Ophthalmology. 2015;**63**(2):103-109

[79] Hayden B, Jockovich ME, Murray TG, et al. Iontophoretic delivery of carboplatin in a murine model of retinoblastoma. Investigative Ophthalmology & Visual Science. 2006;**47**(9):3717-3721

[80] Martin NE, Kim JW, Abramson DH. Fibrin sealant for retinoblastoma: Where are we? Journal of Ocular Pharmacology and Therapeutics. 2008;**24**(5):433-438. DOI: 10.1089/jop.2007.0110

[81] Kang SJ, Durairaj C, Kompella UB, O'Brien JM, Grossniklaus HE. Subconjunctival nanoparticle carboplatin in the treatment of murine retinoblastoma. Archives of Ophthalmology. 2009;**127**(8):1043-1047. DOI: 10.1001/archophthalmol.2009.185

[82] Marr BP, Dunkel IJ, Linker A, Abramson DH. Periocular carboplatin for retinoblastoma: Long-term report (12 years) on efficacy and toxicity. The British Journal of Ophthalmology. 2012;**96**(6):881-883. DOI: 10.1136/bjophthalmol-2011-300517

[83] Mulvihill A, Budning A, Jay V, et al. Ocular motility changes after subtenon carboplatin chemotherapy for retinoblastoma. Archives of Ophthalmology. 2003;**121**(8):1120-1124. DOI: 10.1001/archopht.121.8.1120

[84] Yousef YA, Halliday W, Chan HS, Héon E, Gallie BL, Dimaras H. No ocular motility complications after subtenon topotecan with fibrin sealant for retinoblastoma. Canadian Journal of Ophthalmology. 2013;**48**(6):524-528. DOI: 10.1016/j.jcjo.2013.05.018

Chapter 7

Histopathological Characteristics and Classification for Prognostic Indicators

Heba Alsharif, Hala Helmi and Azza Maktabi

Abstract

Retinoblastoma (RB) is the most common intraocular tumor in children. It arises from the nuclear layer of the retina, with different growth patterns: endophytic, exophytic, and mixed. Retinoblastoma also has characteristic histopathological appearance with areas of viable tumor, necrosis, and calcifications. The tumor differentiation can be determined by the presence of rosettes—Flexner-Wintersteiner rosettes as well as fleurettes—and tends to become less differentiated with age. Histopathological risk factors are used as prognostic indicators and will be discussed in this chapter together with the typical tissue diagnostic features. These will include optic nerve/choroidal invasion, extraocular extension, and anterior segment involvement. Other prognostic factors with less impact will be discussed as well including the amount of necrosis, mitotic figures, and grading of anaplasia. Furthermore, we will briefly discuss different regression patterns and posttreatment findings in enucleated globes.

Keywords: retinoblastoma, pathological prognostic indicators, optic nerve invasion, choroidal invasion, pathological classification

1. Introduction

Retinoblastoma was first ever described by Petras Pawius from Amsterdam in 1597, and it wasn't until 1809 when James Wardrop of Edinburgh established its origination from the retina and recommended enucleation as a primary treatment method for saving lives [1–3]. Nine years later, the first case of fungus hematodes, old name of retinoblastoma, was reported in the American literature [2, 4]. In the following three decades when the microscope was introduced, Virchow, the well-known pathologist, claimed that this tumor is a glioma as it arises from glial cells [2, 5]. Nevertheless, both the pathologist Simon Flexner (1891) and ophthalmologist Hugo Wintersteiner (1897) believed independently that this tumor is actually a neuroepithelioma due to the presence of cellular rosettes harboring a central lumen histologically. In fact, the Flexner-Wintersteiner rosettes that are diagnostic for retinoblastoma are named after these two physicians [2, 6, 7]. Later in the nineteenth century, the American pathologist Verhoeff confirmed that undifferentiated retinal cells are the original nidus of this tumor; thus, he called it retinoblastoma. This term was first adopted by the American Ophthalmology Society in 1926, and it has been in use since then [2, 8].

2. Gross pathology

The first step of grossing an enucleated eye in preparation for histopathological microscopic examination is establishing the laterality. Several anatomical landmarks provide useful cues to orient the globe properly, and these include the cornea, oblique muscles, and ciliary arteries. The corneal horizontal diameter is larger than its vertical diameter by around 1 mm, and this produces an oval shape (**Figure 1A**). The insertion of the superior oblique muscle tendon after originating from the trochlea is in the superior outer (temporal) quadrant just behind the insertion of the superior rectus muscle tendon. The inferior outer (temporal) quadrant receives the insertion of inferior oblique muscle, just lateral to the optic nerve (**Figure 1B**). Locating the horizontal planes can be done affirmatively by identifying the long posterior ciliary arteries that run horizontally at 3 and 9 o'clock [9].

In the past, the enucleated eye was grossed and processed to produce one pupil-optic nerve (PO) section, which is then studied histopathologically. This practice was abandoned following the consensus of the International Retinoblastoma Staging Working Group (IRSWG) in 2009 where the efforts of 85 members from

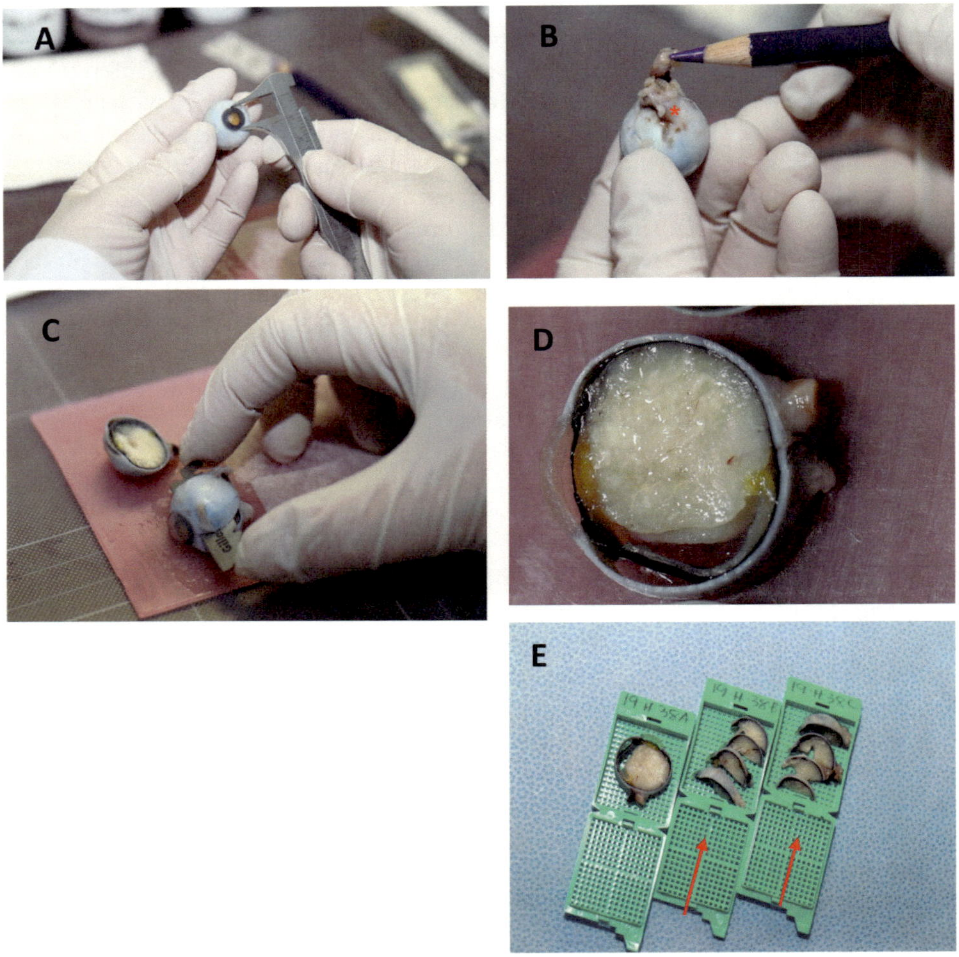

Figure 1.
Grossing an enucleated eye with retinoblastoma: (A) vertical corneal measurements; (B) inferior oblique muscle insertion located temporal (lateral) to the optic nerve (asterisk); (C, D) pupil-optic nerve (PO) section; (E) cassettes containing both calottes cut in bread-loaf pattern (red arrows), while the PO section is submitted in a separate cassette.

24 different countries were joined to establish guidelines for tissue processing and handlining as well as staging. They concluded that the entire enucleated globe should be examined microscopically. This can be achieved by dividing the eye into four blocks. The optic nerve, tumor, and anterior chamber structures are included in the central pupil-optic nerve (PO) section composing one block as demonstrated in (**Figure 1C, D**). Two mirrored blocks composed of the calottes, representing the remaining eye tissue after harvesting the PO section, are usually cut consecutively in a bread-loaf fashion and embedded on edge to increase the examined surface area of the choroid, and this will subsequently improve the chances of detection of choroidal involvement (**Figure 1E**). The last block comprises the optic nerve margin cross section, and this is usually taken initially before cutting the eye. The optic nerve head, lamina cribrosa, and optic nerve posterior to the lamina cribrosa in a single section plane are usually displayed in the PO section as shown in (**Figure 1D**) [9].

Enucleation of the eye not only enables histopathological diagnosis, but it also yields fresh ocular tissue on which molecular and genetic testing can be carried out. Such tests are of paramount importance as their results are needed for family counseling and prognosis prediction. To facilitate this, guidelines and protocols were proposed to ensure preservation of the harvested ocular tissue for examination to obtain the best histopathological and molecular testing results. This guideline states that the enucleated globe should be processed and opened soon after surgery in order to prevent proteins and nucleic acid denaturation. Then, the optic nerve length is measured and documented in mm, and this is followed by preparing the block of the optic nerve margin cut section before proceeding with opening the eye. The next step involves opening the globe with the aid of transillumination, which is helpful in localizing the margins of the intraocular mass in addition to planning the collection of the PO section. Opening the eye can be accomplished using one of two techniques. The first proposed technique involves creating a window opening in the sclera adjacent to the edge of the bulk of the tumor. This scleral window is ideally created using a trephine. The second method is done utilizing a large bore 22-gauge needle that is used under sterile conditions to aspirate fresh tumor cells/tissue. The needle is inserted obliquely under direct visualization via the sclera into the posterior chamber behind the lens, and aspiration takes place once it is inside the tumor mass. Finally, the globe is fixed in an adequate amount of formalin for a minimum of 48 hours [10].

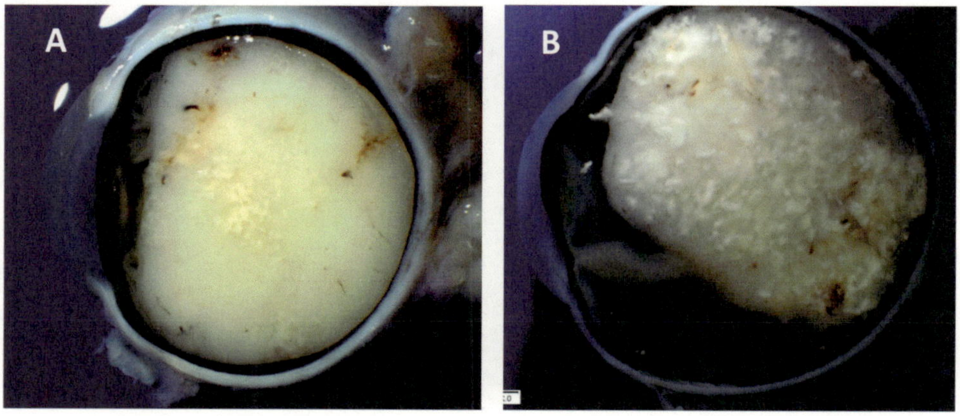

Figure 2.
(A) Gross photo showing the encephaloid appearance of the tumor. (B) White flecks representing the calcification.

Macroscopically, the tumor has an encephaloid appearance, and this is not surprising given that it arises from the retina which resembles the neurological tissue (**Figure 2A**). The tumor is typically white in color, and it encompasses lightly colored flecks. In fact, these flecks are analogous to the dystrophic calcification within the necrotic tissue microscopically (**Figure 2A**) [10].

3. Histopathology

3.1 Tumor origin

Embryologically, retinoblastoma tumors initiate from the inner layer of the optic cup that is derived from the neuroectoderm which is a neurological tissue. At the cellular level, the retinoblastoma constituent cells appear as small, roundish blue cells. Retinal differentiation in RB is categorized as the following: differentiated, undifferentiated, or necrotic. Differentiated tumors are furtherly subdivided into (1) "fleurettes" exhibiting advanced photoreceptor differentiation, (2) the classic Flexner-Wintersteiner rosettes representing early retinal differentiation, (3) Homer Wright rosettes with primitive neuroblastic differentiation, or (4) poorly differentiated [11]. These rosettes in an ascending order of differentiation include Homer Wright, Flexner-Wintersteiner rosettes, and fleurettes providing examples of these histologic structures (**Figure 3**) [2, 10, 12–14]. The Flexner-Wintersteiner rosettes when examined by high magnification microscopy demonstrate a ring of nuclei surrounding a central clear lumen corresponding to the subretinal space (**Figure 3A**). In comparison, the Homer Wright rosettes surround a central tangle of neural filaments with no clear distinct lumen (**Figure 3A**) [10, 11]. The different types of rosettes and/or fleurettes (**Figure 3B**) observed in RB tumors represent varying degrees of differentiation, and these are recognized based on the histologic architectural pattern.

3.2 General histopathology

On microscopic examination, the neuroblastic tumor cells are mitotically active with scanty cytoplasm and irregular basophilic nuclei. Apoptosis leading to necrosis

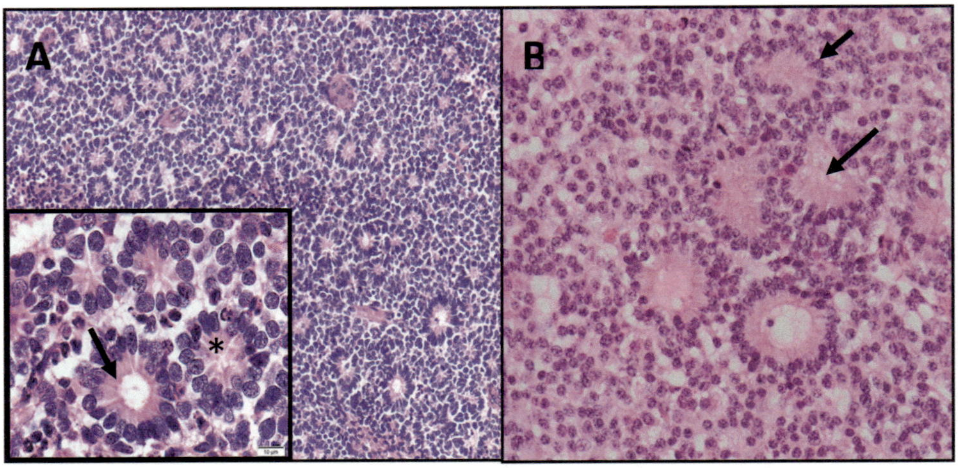

Figure 3.
(A) Different types of rosettes noted by low power. High-power slide showing two types of rosettes: Flexner-Wintersteiner rosettes (arrow) and Homer Wright rosettes (asterisk). (B) Bland-looking pinkish tumor cells with fleurettes (arrow) (original magnification ×1000 stained with hematoxylin and eosin).

is also frequently seen in these tumors. Necrotic areas may develop dystrophic calcification which is the source of the red purple color seen on sections stained with the hematoxylin and eosin (H&E) stain (**Figure 4**) [2, 10, 15]. These calcifications are of great clinical value, and they are usually detected by B-scan ultrasonography.

The level of differentiation of these cells varies, and there is a negative correlation between advancing age and the level of differentiation (less differentiation in older children). Notably, an inverse relationship was detected between retinal differentiation and age, where older infants present with poorer retinal differentiation than young infants in whom microscopic examination of their enucleated eyes revealed good differentiation with the presence of Flexner-Wintersteiner rosettes [11, 16].

Histopathological examination of removed tumors showed that one-fifth of the cases have foci of differentiated photoreceptors. This condition is attributed to a lesser degree of apoptosis and cellular turnover in highly differentiated tumors as photoreceptor differentiation, which persist regardless of the age, unlike Flexner-Wintersteiner rosettes, which were noted to decrease with older age [10, 11]. It was hypothesized that retinoblastomas originate from retinomas or retinocytomas, which are benign tumors entirely formed of differentiated photoreceptors and what proves this theory is the presence of well-differentiated photoreceptor foci at the base of endophytic retinoblastomas. Moreover, Dimaras demonstrated the presence of both RB1 gene mutation in these benignly behaving precursor tumors mentioned above [10, 17].

3.3 High-risk histopathological features

Detecting the presence of high-risk features on histopathological examination is of utmost significance. This is because of the implications these factors have on the risk of systemic metastasis and overall survival. Moreover, the presence of these factors dictates the institution of post-enucleation systemic chemotherapy to improve survival rates and limit the risk of metastasis [9, 11, 18–22].

Several studies from different parts of the world attempted to identify and evaluate these high-risk factors that include the following: retrolaminar optic nerve invasion (**Figure 5**), massive choroidal invasion (**Figures 6** and 7), anterior segment tumor invasion, and extraocular/extra-scleral tumor extension (**Figure 8**) [9, 11, 18–20, 23].

Optic nerve invasion is usually classified as prelaminar (anterior the lamina cribrosa), laminar (involving the lamina cribrosa but not extending beyond it), retrolaminar (extending beyond the lamina cribrosa), and tumor at the surgical cut margin (**Figure 5A–C**). In addition to the length of invasion, the focus of tumor

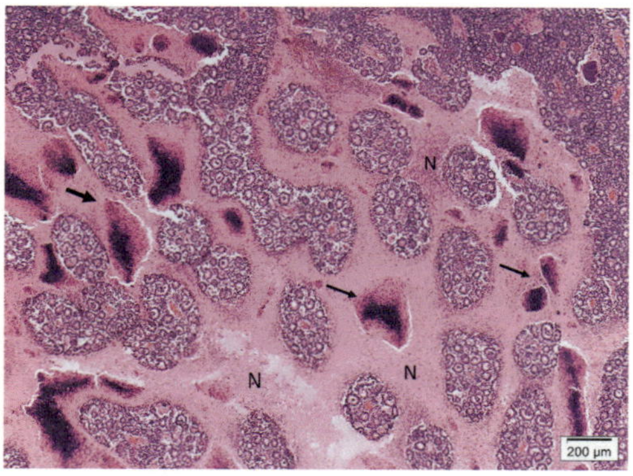

Figure 4.
Low-power histopathological appearance of the tumor demonstrating pseudorosettes. Note the extensive necrosis (N) and calcification (arrow) (original magnification ×40 hematoxylin and eosin).

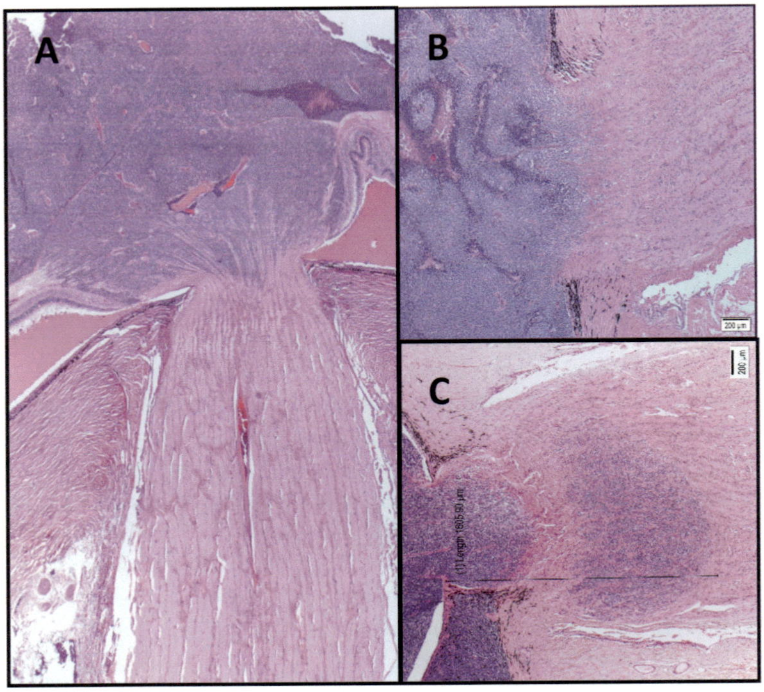

Figure 5.
Histopathological photos of several retinoblastoma tumors showing various degrees of optic nerve invasion: (A) prelaminar, (B) intralaminar, and (C) postlaminar, measuring the depth from Bruch's membrane (hematoxylin and eosin ×40).

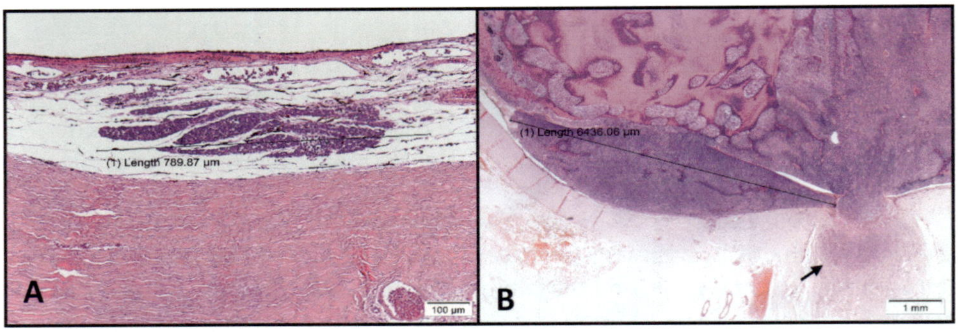

Figure 6.
(A) Microscopic photos showing focal choroidal invasion <3 mm, (hematoxylin and eosin ×100). (B) Massive choroidal invasion>3 mm, (hematoxylin and eosin ×12.5). Note the postlaminar optic nerve invasion (arrow).

invasion must be determined by measuring the maximum depth of invasion into the optic nerve. This is achieved by measuring from the internal limiting membrane (ILM) of the optic disc or Bruch's membrane if ILM was destroyed by the tumor to the deepest area of invasion as demonstrated in (**Figure 5C**) [24, 25]. On the other hand, experts defined massive as more than 3 mm foci of choroidal invasion whether in thickness or width, whereas focal choroidal invasion was defined as less than 3 mm foci of choroidal invasion whether in thickness or width (**Figures 6** and 7). Another helpful anatomical definition is whether the tumor cells are reaching the inner scleral layers in massive invasion or not reaching the sclera in focal invasion [9, 11, 18, 19, 26]. It is important not to misinterpret artificial tumor seeding of the choroid or other ocular structures as invasion. This will prevent over-reporting of high-risk features (such as choroidal invasion) and will consequently avoid additional

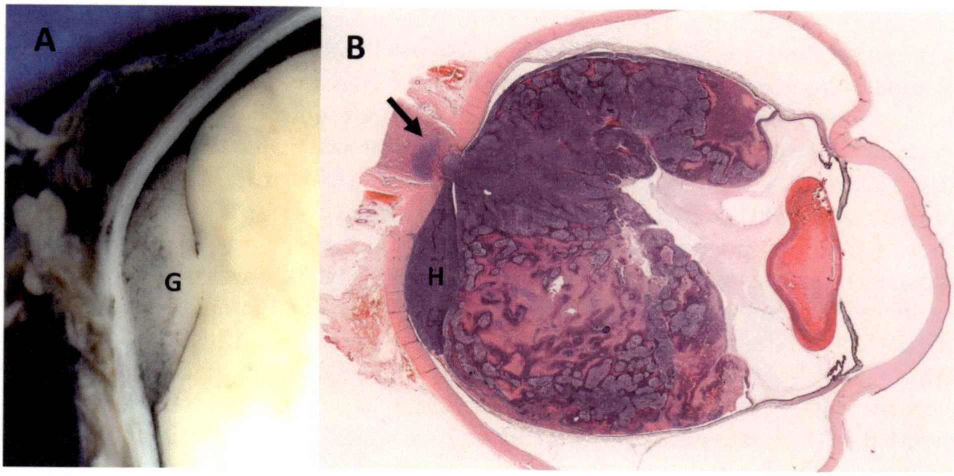

Figure 7.
(A) Massive choroidal invasion noted grossly (G). (B) Corresponding histopathology massive choroidal invasion (H). Note the postlaminar optic nerve invasion (arrow) (hematoxylin and eosin, scanned slide).

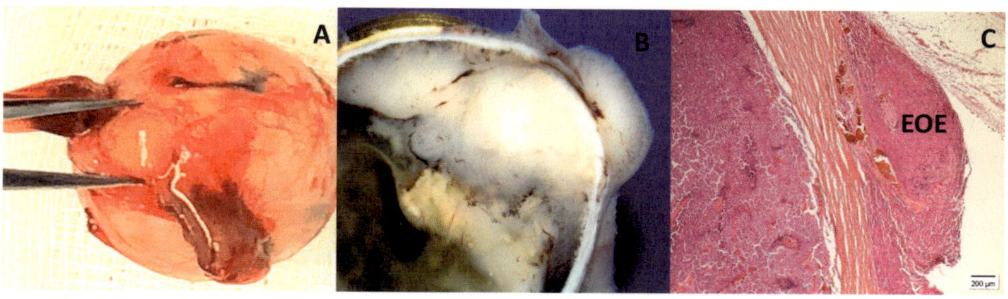

Figure 8.
Extraocular extension identified during surgery (A), grossing (B), and by microscopy (C). Note tumor cells on the outer surface of the sclera (EOE, hematoxylin and eosin ×40).

unnecessary treatments in these vulnerable children. Artificial seeding classically consists of tumor cells clustered in small groups along with many necrotic cells in natural or potential ocular spaces (e.g., suprachoroidal space, anterior chamber, or subarachnoid space of the optic nerve), sectioning artifacts created during tissue preparation and/or ocular surfaces (e.g., episclera, optic nerve meningeal sheath). On the other hand, truly existent invasion consists of solid nests of infiltrative tumor cells that anatomically destroy and substitute the area of invasion; however, necrosis is rarely seen except if the tumor is massive [9, 10].

In the literature, there are several key studies that looked at these high-risk factors. A large study conducted by Eagle et al. from the USA looked at the overall occurrence of high-risk features in children with unilateral retinoblastoma (n = 387), whether treated preoperatively or not, and found an incidence of 20.4%. Further evaluation of the untreated group (n = 297) revealed that high-risk features were present in 18.5% of the enucleated eyes. Among these, retrolaminar optic nerve invasion was the commonest feature occurring in 10.4% followed by massive choroidal invasion in 8.1%, and lastly a combination of both features was observed in 3.4% [11]. In fact, these percentages were similar to those (11.6 and 9.3% for retrolaminar optic nerve invasion and massive uveal invasion, respectively) reported previously by large specialized American treatment centers [11, 27]. The incidence of high-risk features is to the lower side in developed countries (e.g., 20% in the USA); yet, higher rates were observed in developing countries ranging between 29 and 48% [28, 29]. Gupta studied retrospectively 142 cases of retinoblastoma eye enucleated over a 5-year period and found that the high-risk histopathologic features were present in 54.2% of these eyes. Choroidal invasion was the most frequent where it was detected in 40% followed by retrolaminar optic nerve invasion 17% and less commonly other ocular structures such as the iris and sclera. This study further linked the identified high-risk features to the clinical presentation and reported a positive correlation between age > 24 months and choroidal invasion, whereas iris neovascularization correlated with both retrolaminar optic nerve invasion and choroidal invasion [11, 18]. Furthermore, Kaliki evaluated patients with an International Classification of Retinoblastoma (ICRB) classes D and E for high-risk features and reported their presence in 17% of class D eyes (15/87) and 24% of class E eyes (102/432). The fact that high-risk features were more likely to be present in advanced disease is evidently supported by the fact that 10% of patients demonstrating high-risk features on histopathology in the previous study developed metastasis which was fatal in two children. To compare, none of the children in group D with high-risk features developed metastasis nor died [19].

Overall, choroidal and optic nerve invasion reported incidences in the literature are variable and were noticed to be higher in previous publication than more recent ones [23, 28, 30–34]. To add, a trend of higher occurrence was observed in developing countries and specific geographic locations such as Asia and India, and this is explained by the later presentation and unique biological behavior of tumors in these areas. This variability in incidence was looked at by Eagle where he attributed it to multiple factors including diagnosis to enucleation time, reporting institute location and ununified assessing techniques of enucleating specimens [11].

The survival rates in the presence of these high-risk features are usually decreased. In general, patients with massive choroidal invasion had a 70% survival rate, while patients with tumor extending up to the optic nerve cut margin had an obviously lower survival rate of approximately 35%. On the contrary, those with prelaminar optic nerve invasion had excellent survival rates reaching more than 90% [2, 24, 35].

3.4 Other histopathological features

3.4.1 Necrosis

Another characteristic feature seen in RB cases is tumor or ocular tissue necrosis. This condition occurs secondary to mitotically active tumor cells that grow 90–110 micron from the tumor-feeding vessels resulting in ischemia and necrosis. Papillary appearance may be seen in necrotic tissue termed as pseudorosettes (wrong nomenclature) consisting of basophilic viable tissue resembling sleeves and cuffs measuring 100um from the central blood vessels separated by eosinophilic necrotic sheets (**Figure 9**) [10, 15, 20].

Chong studied the association between extensive tumor and ocular tissue necrosis in RB enucleated eyes with high-risk histopathological features. Extensive tissue necrosis was defined as more than 95% of ocular tissue or tumor to be necrotic in enucleated samples. The total number of eyes showing extensive necrosis is 11 (25.6%) out of 43 enucleated eyes. Histopathological high-risk features were more prevalent and statistically significant in enucleated eyes with extensive necrosis. On review of histopathological slides, 11 (100%) had optic nerve invasion with 8 (72.2%) showing retrolaminar invasion and 9 (81.8%) with choroidal invasion. This study concluded that the presence of extensive necrosis of tumor or ocular tissue in

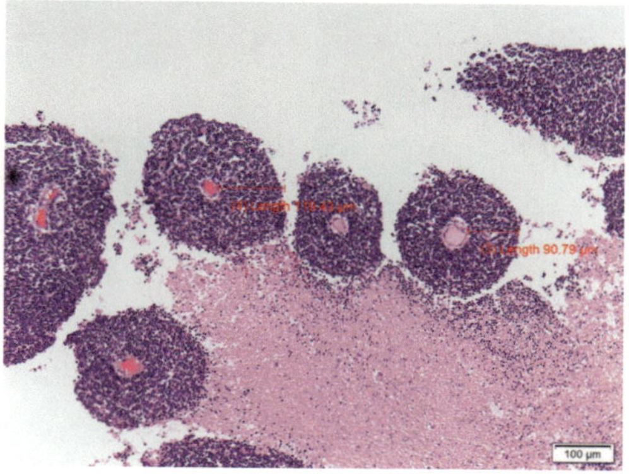

Figure 9.
Pseudorosettes with viable blue cell tumor survived for about 100 um from the central blood vessels, surrounded by pink necrotic tissue.

RB should alert the ocular pathologist to extensively review the slides for high-risk histopathological features to improve the survival rate and lower the risk of metastasis [20].

3.4.2 Growth pattern

RB originates and destroys the neurosensory retina. The tumor is subdivided into two types based on the growth pattern. Endophytic tumors, which are known to be the most common type, arise from the inner layers of the retina which maintains its attachment and normally invades into the vitreous chamber (**Figure 10C, D**) [10]. They are clinically visible by ophthalmoscopy as white mass lesions surrounded by fine feeding vessels, which may be mistaken for an astrocytic hamartoma [36]. These tumors may also occasionally seed the anterior chamber. On the other hand, exophytic tumors arise from the outer retinal layers in between the sensory retina and the retinal pigment epithelium and grow outward typically causing high bullous retinal detachments which may progress to total retinal detachment (**Figure 10A, B**) [10, 36]. They are usually invisible by ophthalmoscopy but may initially be identified with difficulty as small gray masses [36]. They may also cause anterior displacement of the lens-iris diaphragm and secondary angle closure [10]. When presenting with a total retinal detachment, exophytic tumors may be mistaken as Coats disease, persistent hyperplastic primary vitreous, retinopathy of prematurity, or retinal dysplasia [36]. The two previously mentioned growth patterns may overlap manifesting as a mixed endophytic-exophytic retinoblastoma [10]. Rarely, a diffuse infiltrating RB may be found which grows diffusely within the retina without forming a discrete mass. These usually present with signs suggestive of inflammation and are misdiagnosed as uveitis [36].

In 1990, Palazzi classified 297 cases of RB into two types of growth pattern. Their study showed that 61% of the cases were endophytic, while 39% of the cases were exophytic [37]. Similarly, in a more recent study published in 2014, Nawaiseh reported 42 cases of RB where 45% of cases were endophytic, 33% were exophytic, and 21% were mixed endophytic-exophytic. The study did not report any cases of the diffuse infiltrating type [36]. However, Taktikos reported the diffuse infiltrating type in 1% of the cases in his published article in 1966 [38].

The growth patterns have different impacts on the pathological features of the tumor in the eyes with retinoblastoma and no treatment prior to enucleation. Endophytic tumors, which have a direct contact with the vitreous, are more likely

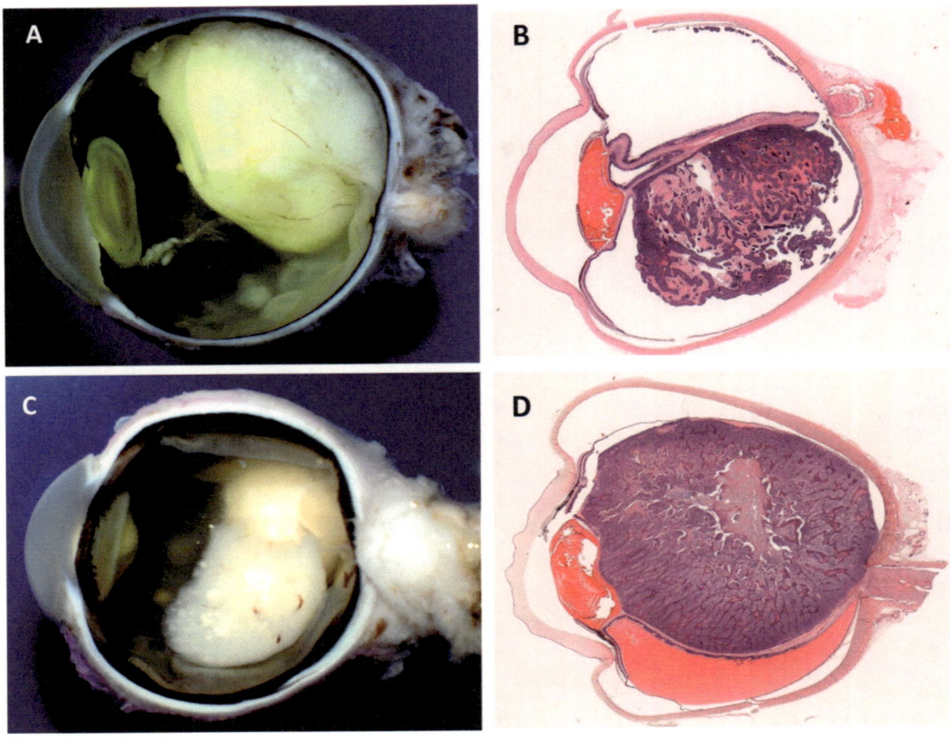

Figure 10.
(A) Gross photo of an exophytic growth pattern (posterior to the retina). (B) Low magnification sample demonstrating exophytic growth pattern (hematoxylin and eosin). (C) Gross photo of an endophytic growth pattern (anterior to the retina) with subretinal fluid. (D) Low magnification sample demonstrating endophytic growth pattern with subretinal fluid (hematoxylin and eosin).

to be associated with vitreous seeds than exophytic tumors. On the other hand, exophytic tumors characteristically grow toward the choroid with a higher risk of choroidal invasion than endophytic tumors. This theory was supported by Palazzi's findings where 71% of tumors with choroidal invasion had an exophytic growth pattern [37]. Nawaiseh also found that all cases with massive choroidal invasion occurred with tumors of exophytic growth patterns [36].

3.5 Correlation between clinical classifications and the high-risk pathological features

Wilson and Kaliki found that group Vb eyes according to the Reese-Ellsworth (RE) classification (eyes with vitreous seeds) have higher incidence of high-risk features than group Va (eyes without vitreous seeds) [19, 39, 40]. The risk of optic nerve invasion (laminar or postlaminar) was found to be 58% in that group, while the risk of massive choroid invasion was as low as 29% [39]. Nawaiseh correlated the above conclusions by Wilson to his own findings and anticipated that endophytic tumors are more likely to be associated with optic nerve invasion rather than choroidal invasion based on the fact that vitreous seeding was more likely to be associated with an endophytic growth pattern [36].

A mixed tumor growth pattern indicated a more advanced tumor stage and a more damaging tumor. Nawaiseh found that the mixed tumor growth pattern was more likely to be associated with neovascular glaucoma and with more advanced IIRC groups (67% were associated with IIRC group E, the most advanced stage of intraocular RB) [36]. On the other hand, Palazzi found that neovascular glaucoma was more likely to be associated with the exophytic tumor which may be due to the long-standing retinal detachment leading to ischemia. However, in that study, only the exophytic and endophytic growth patterns were studied without the mixed growth pattern [37].

3.6 Histopathology of retinoblastoma in enucleated globes following treatment

The well-differentiated part of the RB is relatively radioresistant and chemoresistant; therefore, photoreceptor differentiation is more common in the enucleated eyes after radiotherapy or chemotherapy [11].

The histopathological examination of the enucleated eyes with RB after chemoreduction therapy may show Type 1, cottage cheese; Type 2, fish flesh; Type 3, combination of types 1 and 2; and Type 4, complete regression or presumably viable histologically intact tumor cells [3, 41, 42]. Type 2 regression pattern may have the same histological features as a retinocytoma and result in a retinocytoma-like clinical appearance, which may be because well-differentiated tumors are relatively resistant to chemotherapy and therefore the cells are not cycling [42]. Similar regression patterns are also seen in tumors treated by intra-arterial chemotherapy (IAC) [43].

4. American Joint Committee on Cancer (AJCC) classification

The American Joint Committee on Cancer and the International Union Against Cancer (AJCC/UICC) created a TNM staging scheme system for RB [26, 44–46]. It has multiple updated editions where the 8th edition is the latest updated one [45]. It is considered one of the extraocular classification systems besides the International Retinoblastoma Staging System (IRSS) [47]. Unlike other staging systems, TNM and IRSS were developed by multiple specialists and medical centers worldwide [48, 49]. The TNM8 system is subclassified into clinical, pathological, and hereditary classifications which stand for cTNM, pTNM, and H, respectively [45]. Furthermore, pathological staging necessitates enucleation of the eye to classify primary tumor plus examining local extension or distant metastasis by biopsies or total resection if present. The pTNM categories are divided to pT, the histological staging of the primary tumor after biopsy or enucleation, pN stands for microscopic examination of lymph node biopsy, and clinical plus microscopic examination of distant metastatic lesions implies as M [45, 49]. However, on initial evaluation application of clinical or cTNM, subclassification is wildly used by ophthalmologist which subclassify the tumor burden to intraretinal, intraocular, advanced intraocular, or extraocular [47]. The clinical "cTNM" and hereditary "H" classification are beyond the scope of this chapter. Further details of pTNM classification and staging are demonstrated in **Table 1** [45].

The updated pathological TNM8 version emphasized the importance to define focal, massive choroidal invasion and scleral invasion in compression to previously published TNM7 and TNM6 staging system in 2009 and 2002, respectively [45, 46, 49]. Furthermore, newly updated TNM8 staging system officially released formal staging group for prognosis. It is subdivided into four stages assigned for both clinical and pathological classifications as seen in **Table 1** [45]. Guillermo reported poor disease-free survival in patients staged by the pTNM7 staging system due to omission of scleral invasion. The major event of disease-free survival was extraocular relapse [49].

Pathological classification (pTNM)	
Definition of primary tumor (pT)	
pT Categoery	pT Criteria
pTX	Unknow evidence of intraocular tumor
pT0	No evidence of intraocular tumor
pT1	Intraocular tumor(s) without any local invasion, focal choroidal invasion, or pre- or intralaminar involvement of the optic nerve head
pT2	Intraocular tumor(s) with local invasion
pT2a	Concomitant focal choroidal invasion and pre- or intralaminar involvement of the optic nerve head
pT2b	Tumor invasion of stroma of iris and/or trabecular meshwork and/or Schlemm's canal
pT3	Intraocular tumor(s) with significant local invasion
pT3a	Massive choroidal invasion (>3mm in largest diameter, or multiple foci of focal choroidal involvement totaling >3mm, or any full thickness choroidal involvement)
pT3b	Retrolaminar invasion of the optic nerve head not involving the transected end of the optic nerve
pT3c	Any partial thickness involvement of the sclera within the inner two thirds
pT3d	Full thickness invasion into the outer third of the sclera and/or invasion into or around the emissary channels
pT4	Evidence of extraocular tumor: tumor at the trasected end of optic nerve, tumor in the meningeal spaces around the optic nerve, full thickness invasion of the sclera with the invasion of episclera, adjacent adipose tissue, extraocular muscle, bone, conjunctiva, or eyelids
Definition of Regional Lmyph node (pN)	
pN Category	pN Criteria
pNX	Regional lymph node involvement cannot be assessed
pN0	No lymph node involvement
pN1	Regional lymph node involvement
Definition of distant metastasis (M)	
M Category	M Criteria
cM0	No signs or symptoms of intracranial or distant metastasis
cM1	Distant metastasis without microscopic confirmation
cM1a	Tumor(s) involving any distant site (bone marrow, liver) on clinical or radiological tests
cM1b	Tumor involving the CNS on radiological imaging (not including trilateral retinoblastoma)
pM1	Distant metastasis with histopathological confirmation
pM1a	Histopathological confirmation of tumor at any distant site (bone marrow, liver or other)
pM2	Histopathological confirmation of tumor in the cerebrospinal fluid or CNS parenchyma

AJCC prognostic stages Pathological stage (pTNM)				
pT	**pN**	**M**	**H**	**The pathological stage group**
pT1, pT2, pT3	pN0	cM0	Any	Stage I
pT4	pN0	cM0	Any	Stage II
Any	pN1	cM0	Any	Stage III
Any	Any	cM1 or PM1	Any	Stage IV

Retinoblastoma is a subclassification composed of three aspects: pT, pN, and M. Pathological definition of primary tumor (pT): stands for histopathological staging of the primary tumor after biopsy or enucleation. Pathological definition of lymph node (pN): stands for microscopic examination of lymph node biopsy. Definition of distant metastasis (M): stands for grading distant metastatic lesions including both clinical and pathological definitions.
The abovementioned aspects of pTNM are categorized to 4 stages demonstrated in the last part of **Table 1.**

Table 1.
Pathological TNM classification and staging by the AJCC/UICC for retinoblastoma.

5. Conclusions

Histopathological examination of RB cases is highly valuable in diagnosing, staging, and predicting prognostic factors and risk of metastasis. Further attention should be given while evaluating the four submitted block sections to detect high-risk features that indicate adjuvant chemotherapy administration that lowers metastatic rate and improves the survival rate. The high-risk features include retrolaminar optic nerve invasion, choroidal invasion, anterior chamber involvement, extraocular or extra-scleral spread. Moreover, incidences of previously mentioned high-risk features were studied in various articles. TNM staging created by AJCC/UICC provided pathological staging scheme for retinoblastoma. The recently released 8th edition in 2017 embedded choroidal and scleral invasion definition in tumor pathological staging section. In addition, formal prognostic stages were added.

Acknowledgements

The authors would like to thank the College of Medicine Research Center, Deanship of Scientific Research, King Saud University, and King Khaled Eye Specialist Hospital for their academic support and for providing us with images.

Conflict of interest

There is no financial interest to disclose.

Author details

Heba Alsharif[1], Hala Helmi[2] and Azza Maktabi[3]*

1 Department of Ophthalmology, College of Medicine, King Saud University, Riyadh, Saudi Arabia

2 College of Medicine, Alfaisal University, Riyadh, Saudi Arabia

3 Department of Ophthalmic Pathology/Oncology, King Khaled Eye Specialist Hospital, Riyadh, Saudi Arabia

*Address all correspondence to: az-mak@hotmail.com

References

[1] Pawius P. Observationes anatomical. 1657;**16**:336. Cited by Bartolini, Bartolini Hafniae

[2] Grossniklaus HE. Retinoblastoma. Fifty years of progress. The LXXI Edward Jackson memorial lecture. American Journal of Ophthalmology. 2014;**158**(5):875-891

[3] Bechrakis NE, Bornfeld N, Schueler A, Coupland SE, Henze G, Foerster MH. Clinicopathologic features of retinoblastoma after primary chemoreduction. Archives of Ophthalmology (Chicago, Ill.: 1960). 1998;**116**(7):887-893

[4] Wardrop J. Observations on the Fungus Haematodes or Soft Cancer. Edinburgh: George Ramsay and Co; 2013. p. 1809

[5] Virchow R. Die Krankehaften Geschwulste. Vol. 2. Berlin: August Hirshwald; 1864. pp. 151-169

[6] Flexner S. A peculiar glioma (neuroepithelioma?) of the retina. Bulletin of the Johns Hopkins Hospital. 1891;**2**:115-119

[7] Wintersteiner H. Eine Anatomisfche Und Klinsche Studie. Vienna: Franz Deuticke; 1897. Das Neuroepithleioma Retinae

[8] Verhoeff FH, Jackson E. Minutes of the proceedings, 62nd annual meeting. Transactions of the American Ophthalmological Society. 1926;**24**:38-43

[9] Sastre X, Chantada GL, Doz F, Wilson MW, de Davila MTG, Rodríguez-Galindo C, et al. Proceedings of the consensus meetings from the international retinoblastoma staging working group on the pathology guidelines for the examination of enucleated eyes and evaluation of prognostic risk factors in retinoblastoma. Archives of Pathology & Laboratory Medicine. 2009;**133**(8):1199-1202

[10] Eagle RC. The pathology of ocular cancer. Eye (London, England). 2013;**27**(2):128-136

[11] Eagle RC. High-risk features and tumor differentiation in retinoblastoma: A retrospective histopathologic study. Archives of Pathology & Laboratory Medicine. 2009;**133**(8):1203-1209

[12] Ts'o MO, Zimmerman LE, Fine BS. The nature of retinoblastoma. I. Photoreceptor differentiation: A clinical and histopathologic study. American Journal of Ophthalmology. 1970;**69**(3):339-349

[13] Ts'o MO, Fine BS, Zimmerman LE. The nature of retinoblastoma. II. Photoreceptor differentiation: An electron microscopic study. American Journal of Ophthalmology. 1970;**69**(3):350-359

[14] Bogenmann E, Mark C. Routine growth and differentiation of primary retinoblastoma cells in culture. Journal of the National Cancer Institute. 1983;**70**(1):95-104

[15] Burnier MN, McLean IW, Zimmerman LE, Rosenberg SH. Retinoblastoma. The relationship of proliferating cells to blood vessels. Investigative Ophthalmology & Visual Science. 1990;**31**(10):2037-2040

[16] Madhavan J, Ganesh A, Roy J, Biswas J, Kumaramanickavel G. The relationship between tumor cell differentiation and age at diagnosis in retinoblastoma. Journal of Pediatric Ophthalmology and Strabismus. 2008;**45**(1):22-25

[17] Dimaras H, Khetan V, Halliday W, Orlic M, Prigoda NL, Piovesan B, et al.

Loss of RB1 induces non-proliferative retinoma: Increasing genomic instability correlates with progression to retinoblastoma. Human Molecular Genetics. 2008;**17**(10):1363-1372

[18] Gupta R, Vemuganti GK, Reddy VAP, Honavar SG. Histopathologic risk factors in retinoblastoma in India. Archives of Pathology & Laboratory Medicine. 2009;**133**(8):1210-1214

[19] Kaliki S, Shields CL, Rojanaporn D, Al-Dahmash S, McLaughlin JP, Shields JA, et al. High-risk retinoblastoma based on international classification of retinoblastoma: Analysis of 519 enucleated eyes. Ophthalmology. 2013;**120**(5):997-1003

[20] Chong E-M, Coffee RE, Chintagumpala M, Hurwitz RL, Hurwitz MY, Chévez-Barrios P. Extensively necrotic retinoblastoma is associated with high-risk prognostic factors. Archives of Pathology & Laboratory Medicine. 2006;**130**(11):1669-1672

[21] Honavar SG, Singh AD, Shields CL, Meadows AT, Demirci H, Cater J, et al. Postenucleation adjuvant therapy in high-risk retinoblastoma. Archives of Ophthalmology (Chicago, Ill.: 1960). 2002;**120**(7):923-931

[22] Alkatan HM, ALBalawi H, Maktabi AMY. The value of "en toto" globe submission in the assessment of high-risk retinoblastoma cases and staging. International Ophthalmology. 2018;**38**(1):35-41

[23] Messmer EP, Heinrich T, Höpping W, de Sutter E, Havers W, Sauerwein W. Risk factors for metastases in patients with retinoblastoma. Ophthalmology. 1991;**98**(2):136-141

[24] Chantada GL, Casco F, Fandiño AC, Galli S, Manzitti J, Scopinaro M, et al. Outcome of patients with retinoblastoma and postlaminar optic nerve invasion. Ophthalmology. 2007;**114**(11):2083-2089

[25] Magramm I, Abramson DH, Ellsworth RM. Optic nerve involvement in retinoblastoma. Ophthalmology. 1989;**96**(2):217-222

[26] Mendoza PR, Specht CS, Hubbard GB, Wells JR, Lynn MJ, Zhang Q, et al. Histopathologic grading of anaplasia in retinoblastoma. American Journal of Ophthalmology. 2015;**159**(4):764-776.e3

[27] Uusitalo MS, Van Quill KR, Scott IU, Matthay KK, Murray TG, O'Brien JM. Evaluation of chemoprophylaxis in patients with unilateral retinoblastoma with high-risk features on histopathologic examination. Archives of Ophthalmology (Chicago, Ill.: 1960). 2001;**119**(1):41-48

[28] Biswas J, Das D, Krishnakumar S, Shanmugam MP. Histopathologic analysis of 232 eyes with retinoblastoma conducted in an Indian tertiary-care ophthalmic center. Journal of Pediatric Ophthalmology and Strabismus. 2003;**40**(5):265-267

[29] Chantada GL, Dunkel IJ, de Dávila MTG, Abramson DH. Retinoblastoma patients with high risk ocular pathological features: Who needs adjuvant therapy? The British Journal of Ophthalmology. 2004;**88**(8):1069-1073

[30] Khelfaoui F, Validire P, Auperin A, Quintana E, Michon J, Pacquement H, et al. Histopathologic risk factors in retinoblastoma: A retrospective study of 172 patients treated in a single institution. Cancer. 1996;**77**(6):1206-1213

[31] Kopelman JE, McLean IW, Rosenberg SH. Multivariate analysis of risk factors for metastasis in retinoblastoma treated by enucleation. Ophthalmology. 1987;**94**(4):371-377

[32] Carbajal UM. Metastasis in retinoblastoma. American Journal of Ophthalmology. 1959;**48**(1):47-49

[33] Redler LD, Ellsworth RM. Prognostic importance of choroidal invasion in retinoblastoma. Archives of Ophthalmology (Chicago, Ill.: 1960). 1973;**90**(4):294-296

[34] Shields CL, Shields JA, Baez KA, Cater J, De Potter PV. Choroidal invasion of retinoblastoma: Metastatic potential and clinical risk factors. The British Journal of Ophthalmology. 1993;**77**(9):544-548

[35] Magramm I, Abramson DH, Ellsworth RM. Optic nerve involvement in retinoblastoma. Ophthalmology. 1989;**96**(2):217-222

[36] Nawaiseh I, Al-Hussaini M, Alhamwi A, Meyar M, Sultan I, Alrawashdeh K, et al. The impact of growth patterns of retinoblastoma (endophytic, exophytic, and mixed patterns). Turk Patoloji Dergisi. 2015;**31**(1):45-50

[37] Palazzi M, Abramson DH, Ellsworth RM. Endophytic vs exophytic unilateral retinoblastoma: Is there any real difference? Journal of Pediatric Ophthalmology and Strabismus. 1990;**27**(5):255-258

[38] Taktikos A. Investigation of retinoblastoma with special reference to histology and prognosis. The British Journal of Ophthalmology. 1966;**50**(5):225-234

[39] Wilson MW, Qaddoumi I, Billups C, Haik BG, Rodriguez-Galindo C. A clinicopathological correlation of 67 eyes primarily enucleated for advanced intraocular retinoblastoma. The British Journal of Ophthalmology. 2011;**95**(4):553-558

[40] Reese AB, Ellsworth RM. The evaluation and current concept of retinoblastoma therapy. Transactions of the American Academy of Ophthalmology and Otolaryngology. 1963;**67**:164-172

[41] Dithmar S, Aabert TM, Grossniklaus HE. Histopathologic changes in retinoblastoma after chemoreduction. Retina (Philadelphia, Pa.). 2000;**20**(1):33-36

[42] Demirci H, Eagle RC, Shields CL, Shields JA. Histopathologic findings in eyes with retinoblastoma treated only with chemoreduction. Archives of Ophthalmology (Chicago, Ill.: 1960). 2003;**121**(8):1125-1131

[43] Vajzovic LM, Murray TG, Aziz-Sultan MA, Schefler AC, Fernandes CE, Wolfe SCQ, et al. Clinicopathologic review of enucleated eyes after intra-arterial chemotherapy with melphalan for advanced retinoblastoma. Archives of Ophthalmology (Chicago, Ill.: 1960). 2010;**128**(12):1619-1623

[44] Albert D, Syed N, Cancer Committee, College of American Pathologists. Protocol for the examination of specimens from patients with retinoblastoma: A basis for checklists. Archives of Pathology & Laboratory Medicine. 2001;**125**(9):1183-1188

[45] Mallipatna AC, Gallie BL, Chévez-Barrios P, Lumbroso-Le Rouic L, Chantada G, Doz F, et al. In: Amin MB, Edge SB, Greene FL, et al., editors. AJCC Cancer Staging Manual. 8th ed. New York: Springer; 2017

[46] Edge SB, Byrd DR, Compton CC, Fritz AG, Greene FL, Trotti A, editors. AJCC Cancer Staging Manual. 7th ed. New York: Springer; 2010

[47] Fabian ID, Reddy A, Sagoo MS. Classification and staging of retinoblastoma. Community Eye Health. 2018;**31**(101):11-13

[48] Chantada G, Doz F, Antoneli CBG, Grundy R, Clare Stannard FF, Dunkel IJ, et al. A proposal for an international retinoblastoma staging system. Pediatric Blood & Cancer. 2006;**47**(6):801-805

[49] Chantada GL, Sampor C, Bosaleh A, Solernou V, Fandiño A, de Dávila MTG. Comparison of staging systems for extraocular retinoblastoma: Analysis of 533 patients. JAMA Ophthalmology. 2013;**131**(9):1127-1134

Chapter 8

Secondary Malignancies in Adulthood and after Retinoblastoma Treatment in Childhood

Alena Furdova and Juraj Sekac

Abstract

Advances in retinoblastoma treatment in children nowadays and in the last decades lead to success and adulthood life without problems. Treatment modalities used in childhood to cure the retinoblastoma can affect health later. Some secondary malignancies in patients with retinoblastoma may be long-term side effects of radiation and chemotherapy. However, rates of second cancers in people treated for hereditary retinoblastoma are higher than in people who had sporadic retinoblastoma. The survivors of retinoblastoma in whom second malignant neoplasms develop are at a higher risk for the development of additional tumors than they were for the development of a second tumor. The standardized incidence rate of secondary malignancies is about 15% in inherited cases and about 1.5% in nonheritable retinoblastoma. However, today there is no clear consensus on what, if any, screening protocol would be most appropriate and effective.

Keywords: retinoblastoma, secondary malignancies, secondary tumors after radiotherapy, chemotherapy

1. Retinoblastoma and secondary malignancies

With major advances in retinoblastoma treatment in recent decades, most children treated for retinoblastoma are now expected to have a normal life [1]. Some of the treatment modalities used in childhood to cure the retinoblastoma can affect a child's health later in life, so watching for health effects as they get older has become more of a concern in recent years [2]. The prognosis for survival is excellent. The current therapy includes an improved survival rate and decreased iatrogenic side effects [2–4].

The most common primary intraocular malignant tumor in children is retinoblastoma. Hereditary retinoblastoma with gene Rb1 has bilateral tumor infiltration most frequently. Also children with positive family history are presumed to have a germline Rb1 mutation [3]. Screening of mutations in the Rb1 gene can help to identify heritable retinoblastoma and contribute to clinical management and genetic counseling for affected families [5]. The main criteria in determining the result of a mutation is its location in the 3D structure. The altered 3D model structures of the Rb1 novel mutant proteins are also available today [6, 7].

Improvements in survival, from a 3-year survival rate of 76% in the 1970s to a 5-year survival rate of 97% since the mid-1990s, are due to advances in treatment [2, 8, 9]. But children who survive and have hereditary retinoblastoma have an increased risk for secondary malignant neoplasms (SMN). The most common subsequent malignancies are in bony tissues like sarcomas. Also secondary melanoma can develop most frequently [10, 11]. The authors of several studies in retinoblastoma survivors have reported an increased risk of SMN associated with previous treatment, particularly in radiotherapy (RT) which showed an increased risk when it was indicated in children under the age of 1 year [12–14]. In retinoblastoma survivors increased incidence of common epithelial cancers (especially in the lungs and breast) has been observed [15–18].

Young people treated in childhood for retinoblastoma are at risk, to some degree, for several possible late effects of their cancer treatment. The risk of late effects depends on a number of factors, such as the specific treatments used, the doses of treatment, the type of retinoblastoma (heritable or nonheritable), and the age of the patient when the therapy was used. The late effects of the retinoblastoma treatment are:

- Enucleation of the eye globe leads to loss of vision and cosmetic defects.
- Radiotherapy, especially external radiotherapy, of the affected eye leads to visual acuity loss or reduction and can lead also to deformities of the bony orbit.
- Kidney function reduction.
- Chemotherapy leads to heart problems.
- In children with retinoblastoma, generally, slowed growth and development are observed.
- In children with retinoblastoma generally changes in sexual development and ability to have children are observed.
- In survivors of retinoblastoma in adult age, an increased risk of SMN, especially in children with hereditary retinoblastoma, is present.

2. Secondary cancers after retinoblastoma treatment

Although the risk for a second retinoblastoma decreases significantly after 5 years of age, follow-up on all children after treatment is critical and particularly for those who carry the Rb1 mutation. Retinoblastoma survivors are at increased risk for local secondary complications after treatment, e.g., retinal detachment and cataracts, in later life because of the retinal changes caused by the cancer and therapy modalities. Although the general risk for secondary cancers associated with intravenous chemotherapies is high, it's thought to be lower than the risk from radiation therapy.

2.1 Hereditary retinoblastoma (heritable)

Children with the heritable form of retinoblastoma have a much higher risk of developing other types of cancer throughout their lives. The most common secondary cancers among hereditary retinoblastoma survivors include:

- Osteosarcoma
- Soft tissue sarcomas
- Malignant skin melanoma
- Lung cancer
- Lymphoma
- Bladder cancer
- Uterine cancer
- Breast cancer
- Brain tumors
- Cancers in the head region, mouth, or nose

The risk for these cancers is even higher in any parts of the body that got radiation during treatment for retinoblastoma in childhood. This is because each cell in the body has an abnormal Rb1 tumor suppressor gene, which, if it were normal, would help stop some of these cancers from forming. Most of these cancers are very treatable if detected early, which is why it's very important that these children (young people) are followed closely throughout their lives. Retinoblastoma survivors in adult age have the increased risk of SMN, and it is necessary to teach them and their relatives and speak with them about other factors that might increase their risk of secondary malignancies in adult age. Increased risk of skin melanoma may be due to higher sun exposure, and smoking can increase lung cancer risk. These young survivors have to avoid the risk factors. It is necessary to inform the relatives also about screening tests in adulthood of retinoblastoma survivors.

Children who got the heritable form of retinoblastoma also have a small risk of developing a tumor in the pineal gland within a few years. Magnetic resonance imaging (MRI) scans of the head in retinoblastoma survivors should be done regularly for several years after retinoblastoma treatment in childhood with the aim of detecting secondary tumors as soon as possible.

2.2 Sporadic retinoblastoma (nonheritable)

Patients with the nonheritable form of retinoblastoma who do not have the Rb1 gene change in all of their cells do not have such a high risk of secondary malignancies. Still, the risk of some types of secondary malignancies might be higher as a long-term effect of chemotherapy or external radiation therapy.

2.3 Follow-up

The whole long-life follow-up is necessary to retinoblastoma survivors. Long-term follow-up guidelines for survivors of childhood cancers and also retinoblastoma were invented by the Children's Oncology Group (COG). These guidelines are helpful for relatives but also doctors to send the patient regularly for screening tests, and they help to realize how late effects of, e.g., radiotherapy, can be treated [3].

In child's healthcare team, it is very important to discuss possible long-term complications after treatment and to inform also parents and relatives, if these problems appear, how to treat them. The guidelines of COG are available for healthcare professionals, but also patients' version is available (as "Health Links") on the webpage as well.

2.4 Emotional and social issues

Even though most children with retinoblastoma are very young at the time of diagnosis, under the age of 4, they may have emotional or psychological problems that need to be addressed during the treatment and also after the treatment. Depending on the age of retinoblastoma, these children have some problems at school work due to visual acuity loss or reduction.

The factors can lead to problems in their life and they need help. Doctors, ophthalmologists, oncologists, and other members of the healthcare team like psychologists can recommend special support programs and services to help children during and after treatment and to avoid misdiagnosed secondary malignancies in adulthood. Parents and relatives can also be affected with the situation of primary retinoblastoma treatment and also secondary tumors which appear later. The family situation is worsened; financial stress and traveling to and staying near the cancer center are complicated for the family. Social programs and psychologists can help families deal with these problems. Oncology centers for patients with retinoblastoma may have programs to introduce new patients and their relatives to patients who have finished retinoblastoma therapy.

Loss of visual acuity is serious but enucleation leads to defect in the face. In patients with these problems, social groups and programs for the visually impaired can help. Most children treated for retinoblastoma can have good visual acuity in the unaffected eye, but it can happen that the surrounding tissues around the treated eye and the area of the orbit might have changes and later can lead to secondary malignancies. Such changes can be treated by reconstructive surgery. Early intervention can help to avoid psychological problems and also avoid secondary tumors in soft tissues in the orbit [3].

3. Secondary malignancies

In patients with retinoblastoma, secondary malignancies can be the result of the long-term side effect of radiation and chemotherapy. The incidence of secondary malignancies in children treated for hereditary retinoblastoma is higher than in children with sporadic retinoblastoma. In the study of MacCarthy et al. in 1927, retinoblastoma patients are diagnosed in Britain from 1951 to 2004; standardized incidence rate of secondary malignancies was reported: it was significantly higher in inherited retinoblastoma children—13.7% cases compared to 1.5% in nonheritable cases [19].

Osteosarcoma as the most frequent secondary malignancy following retinoblastoma treatment can be associated with the Rb1 gene and/or induced by radiotherapy. Studies have consistently demonstrated increased risks for bone cancers and soft tissue sarcomas among retinoblastoma survivors who received radiotherapy, but by investigations of chemotherapy, subsequent malignant neoplasm development has been limited. Previous reports among hereditary retinoblastoma survivors in studies have suggested that increased risks of bone cancers and soft tissue sarcomas are associated with chemotherapy [20, 21], but in the study of Wong et al., they were results of first comprehensive analysis of chemotherapy-related SMN risk [22].

In a study of 46 survivors of retinoblastoma who received triethylenemelamine and radiotherapy, 7 secondary malignancies were reported. This malignancies were sarcomas of the bones (femur and orbit), as well as other cancers of the brain, parotid gland, pineal gland, and cervix [23]. In other studies in 18 retinoblastoma survivors who developed a subsequent osteosarcoma, 7 and 6 survivors had received triethylenemelamine or cyclophosphamide, respectively [24].

In retinoblastoma survivors after receiving cyclophosphamide, secondary malignancy as osteosarcoma was frequently reported in other studies [25–27]. In a study of 25 survivors who received RT and developed subsequent soft tissue or bone sarcomas, they received cyclophosphamide, either alone or in combination with other agents [11]. Individual cases of bone cancers have also been reported in patients who received triethylenemelamine [28]. One study reported few secondary malignancies after retinoblastoma treatment with carbocisplatin, vincristine, and etoposide, but the mean follow-up time for hereditary survivors was only up to 7 years [29]. Additional follow-up in the future is needed to capture the typical age groups and intervals after retinoblastoma therapy for adults for SMN development. In a study of 15 retinoblastoma survivors with secondary acute myelogenous leukemia, 12 of them had been treated with adjuvant chemotherapy, including topoisomerase II inhibitors, epipodophyllotoxins, and alkylating agents [30].

Studies of chemotherapy treatment for retinoblastoma and related SMN risks among retinoblastoma survivors are limited. But some results of previous studies reported CT-related risks of bone cancers among childhood cancer survivors. A case-control study of the UK National Registry of Childhood Tumors reported a nonsignificant 2.1-fold increased risk for bone cancers in the chemotherapy plus RT group relative to the group receiving RT only [26]. Childhood cancer survivors who had an alkylator score ≥ 3 and had received irradiation ≥ 1000 rad had a 1.6-fold increased risk for bone cancers as it was reported in another case-control analysis [31]. In both abovementioned studies, a supra-additive effect was observed when comparing the chemotherapy plus RT relative risk with the independent risks for RT and chemotherapy. There was a greater risk when survivors were treated with both as opposed to RT or chemotherapy alone [26, 27, 31]. The result in study of Wong et al. was limited to the small number of retinoblastoma survivors who were treated with chemotherapy but no RT, and there are no reported SMNs in this treatment group. But they were unable to estimate SMN risks associated with CT alone [22]. These studies also demonstrate a positive dose-response relationship for the alkylator score with bone sarcoma risk among childhood cancer survivors treated with chemotherapy only.

In studies among retinoblastoma survivors who received chemotherapy and RT, risk is increased for soft tissue sarcomas, especially leiomyosarcomas. A case-control analysis of a UK-based cohort of childhood cancer survivors reported a positive dose-response relationship for soft tissue sarcoma among survivors treated with alkylating agents [32]. Previous studies among retinoblastoma survivors have reported higher SMN risk with RT administered before the age of 1 year [12, 14, 33]. Although the alkylating agent-related risk estimate for leiomyosarcomas was higher for receipt of alkylating agents at age < 1 than for age ≥ 1 year, this difference was not statistically significant, and thus, it remains unclear whether treatment-related risks differ by age. Further research is needed to understand whether younger individuals may be more susceptible to alkylating agent-related SMNs. Other studies also noted a particularly elevated risk for leiomyosarcomas compared with other soft tissue sarcomas after retinoblastoma treatment, but those studies lacked data on retinoblastoma treatments [7, 15, 30, 31]. Loss of heterozygosity in Rb1 and in other major tumor suppressor genes, as well as deletions of chromosome 13, that contain the Rb1 gene has been reported in individuals who developed uterine leiomyosarcomas. Future genetic studies in this population could elucidate the predisposition for leiomyosarcomas in patients with retinoblastoma [35, 36].

Children with the heritable form of retinoblastoma also have a very small risk to develop within a few years a tumor in the pineal gland; it is referred as a trilateral retinoblastoma. Tumors can start there, while the pineal gland can have cells similar to retina cells. That is why it is important to perform MRI of the head for several years after treatment of retinoblastoma to detect these tumors as early as possible. Trilateral retinoblastoma has been the principal cause of death from retinoblastoma in the United States during the first decade of life [37]. Yamanaka, Hayno, and Takashima analyzed 211 cases of trilateral retinoblastomas. The average latency period between the onset of retinoblastomas and trilateral retinoblastomas was 1.5 ± 1.8 years. Pineal tumors were found in almost 74% and sellar tumors in 22%. The overall median survival was 10.3 months, and the 5-year survival rate was 16%, while in patients receiving high-dose chemotherapy by stem cell transplantation, the survival time was significantly longer than with conventional chemotherapy. The authors conclude that trilateral retinoblastoma patients with an irradiation history had shorter survival than those without irradiation history for retinoblastoma, and high-dose chemotherapy should be considered as a potential treatment option for trilateral retinoblastomas [38].

Among patients with hereditary disease, treatment with radiotherapy in 95% was associated with a further increase in the risk of a subsequent cancer. After 30 years of follow-up, elevated risks of epithelial cancers (lung, bladder, and breast) were observed among survivors of hereditary retinoblastoma [18]. In the study of Wong et al., it was found that the incidence of secondary cancer after retinoblastoma treatment is higher due to the genetic predisposition. Genetic predisposition has a substantial impact on risk of subsequent cancers in retinoblastoma survivors, and radiation treatment increases it. A radiation dose-response relationship is demonstrated in all types of soft tissue sarcomas. Retinoblastoma patients should be examined for new cancers and followed into later life also in whole adulthood due to extraordinary secondary cancer risk [39].

The development of lung cancer is affected to a considerable extent by somatic mutations in the Rb1 gene in patients with an elevated risk for lung cancer. Higher risk of developing lung cancer is in patients undergoing chemotherapy and radiotherapy in retinoblastoma treatment [40, 41]. Some studies suggested there might also be an increased risk for lung cancer in non-irradiated patients [15].

Bladder tumors are distinguished between malignant and nonmalignant. In this case, there is only a small difference between them that is difficult to determine microscopically. The most common bladder cancer is papilloma and papillomavirus, which together account for about 90% of all tumors. The borderline between malignant and nonmalignant bladder tumors is very thin [42]. Study of Marees et al. significantly elevated risk of bladder cancer among hereditary retinoblastoma patients after prolonged follow-up, whose prevalence is mostly 30 years after retinoblastoma treatment [18]. Alterations in an Rb1 pathway have been established as a major contributor to bladder tumorigenesis, and carriers of an Rb1 mutation have an elevated risk of bladder cancer, when they reach the ages at which these malignancies occur in the population at large [43].

All available studies on the occurrence of secondary malignity after retinoblastoma treatment indicate that the most important risk factor remains the Rb1 gene mutation.

Kleinerman describes in his study the risks of new cancers after radiotherapy in long-term survivors of retinoblastoma. Radiation increases the risk of another cancer in hereditary patients by 3.1-fold. Hereditary patients continue to have at significantly increased risk for sarcomas, melanoma, and cancers of the brain and nasal cavities [44].

3.1 Case report 1

Girl with bilateral retinoblastoma treated in 1989 in Bratislava by enucleation of the right eye and chemotherapy plus RT on the left side. Due to secondary complication, she underwent cataract surgery in 1993 and was aphakic and got glasses. In 2011 secondary tumor developed in the orbit region with infiltration to the brain. She underwent surgery three times by a neurosurgeon with adjuvant chemotherapy and high-dose RT due to verified leiomyosarcoma. In 2015 due to progression of the leiomyosarcoma, she underwent photon beam irradiation with gamma knife. Tumor masses infiltrating the orbit lead to exenteration of the orbit (**Figures 1–3**).

The risk of secondary malignancies after retinoblastoma treatment is high, but in contrast to bone cancers and leiomyosarcomas, chemotherapy was not associated with increased melanoma risk [10, 17]. The development of skin melanoma may be related to an underlying genetic predisposition associated with retinoblastoma rather than treatment modality. Major susceptibility genes for melanoma include CDKN2A and CDK4 which are both upstream from the Rb1 gene. In the future an additional investigation is necessary to understand the association between the development of melanoma and retinoblastoma treatment [45].

The leukemogenicity of certain chemotherapeutic agents is well established, and there are connections between alkylating agents and a range of development of solid

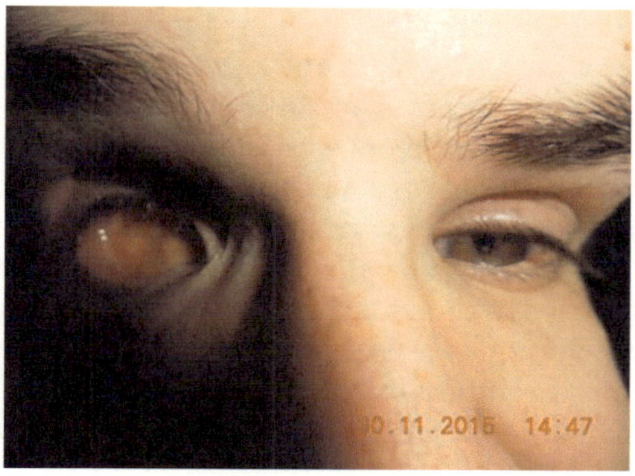

Figure 1.
Case report 1: Patient after enucleation of her right eye in childhood; conjunctival sac clear; in her left eye, aphakia (clinical findings in 2015).

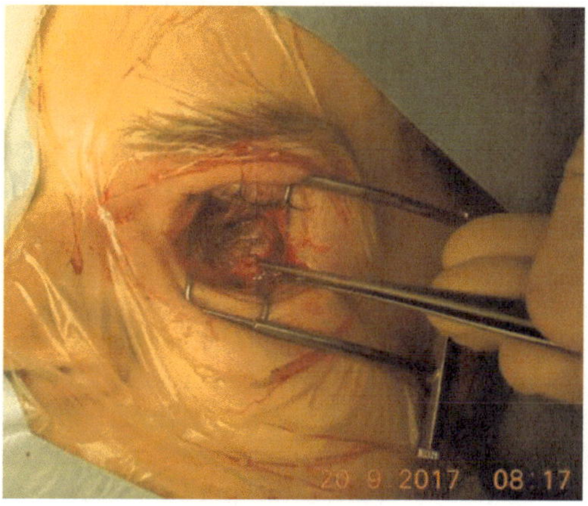

Figure 2.
Case report 1: Preoperative findings in 2017 by partial exenteration of the left orbit due to secondary tumor—Histopathologically confirmed leiomyosarcoma grade 2.

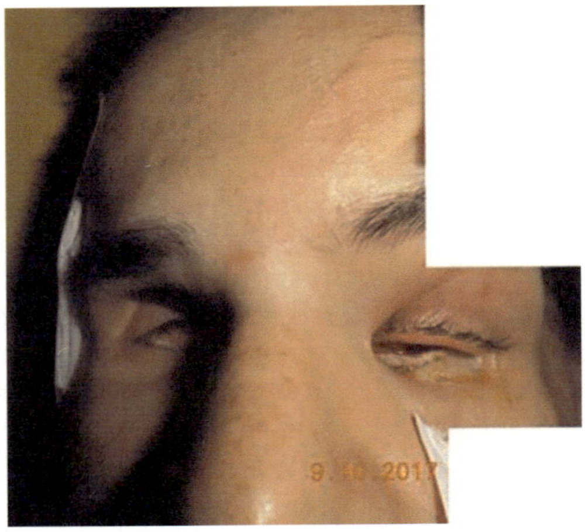

Figure 3.
Case report 1: Clinical findings next month after surgery of the left orbit, healing without complications.

SMNs. Chemotherapy has also been associated with an increased risk for other types of malignancies, e.g., lung cancer after Hodgkin and non-Hodgkin lymphomas, stomach cancer after Hodgkin lymphoma in combination with high-dose abdominal RT, and colorectal cancer after childhood cancer [46, 47]. Increased sarcoma risk after childhood cancer is associated with anthracyclines therapy, especially after Hodgkin lymphoma or a primary sarcoma in childhood [48].

Hereditary retinoblastoma survivors who were treated with alkylating agents plus RT have a significantly higher risk of developing bone cancers and leiomyosarcomas than those treated with single RT. Excess risks of secondary cancers associated with alkylating agents plus RT persist for decades. Significantly higher incidence of leiomyosarcomas is diagnosed at a median age of 34 years. These risks are present during long-term follow-up of retinoblastoma survivors. Guide recommendations for future treatment protocols will define chemo-related SMN risk among retinoblastoma survivors, particularly in patients treated with chemotherapy without RT.

Current chemotherapy agents recommended for retinoblastoma include cyclophosphamide, ifosfamide, carboplatin, vincristine, etoposide, topotecan, and doxorubicin [49–51]. Most retinoblastoma survivors who received an alkylating agent received TEM, which is no longer used in clinical practice [52]. On the basis of the recently developed cyclophosphamide equivalent dose, TEM has substantially lower hematologic toxicity than agents used in current clinical practice. Generally there is the long latency period of SMN development and potentially different CT drug-related adverse effect. In the future studies have to evaluate SMN risk with long-term follow-up of patients with retinoblastoma treated with current agents. The cyclophosphamide equivalent dose can be easily calculated, facilitating its use for patient counseling. It is independent of the drug dose distribution of a particular patient population, a characteristic that will allow direct comparisons of outcomes among epidemiological cohorts. The use of the cyclophosphamide equivalent dose is promising in future research, assessing cumulative alkylating agent exposure [53].

Several limitations of certain studies dealing with SMNs should be taken into account. On reports of family history of retinoblastoma and laterality to define hereditary status, some unilateral retinoblastoma survivors could have had a germline Rb1 mutation and should have been included into analysis [17, 34].

Although some survivors in studies are lost to follow-up due to different reasons, SMN risk estimates are unlikely to be affected, because response was not related to treatment received for retinoblastoma [54]. Due to results of Wong et al., although SMNs are more likely to be misclassified because histology is not specified, sensitivity analyses including 1-year versus 5-year survivors also yielded comparable results [22].

Skin malignancies are rare but usually are in the head region. Orbital malignancies are more frequent. In the study was presented a 22-year-old young man with history of bilateral retinoblastoma initially in childhood treated by enucleation of his left eye. The histopathology findings showed a moderately differentiated tumor with vitreous seeding. The patient received chemotherapy in addition to radiotherapy to his right eye. More than 20 years later, he got proptosis due to the right orbital tumor. The excisional biopsy of his orbital mass verified a spindle cell sarcoma with features of malignant fibrous histiocytoma [55].

3.2 Case report 2

Boy with unilateral retinoblastoma treated in 1988 in Bratislava with enucleation of the left eye globe and chemotherapy and RT. He got individual prosthesis

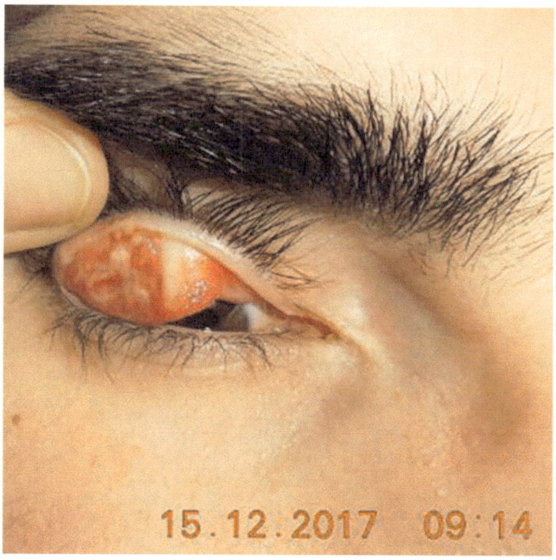

Figure 4.
Case report 2: Secondary tumor in his upper right eye lid (histopathologically confirmed squamous cell carcinoma of the eyelid).

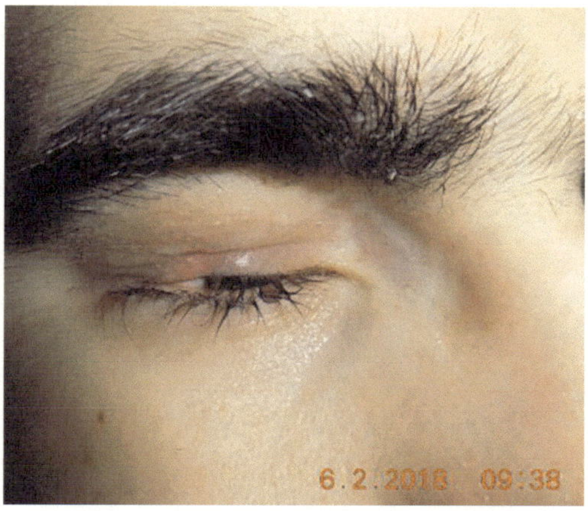

Figure 5.
Case report 2: Patient 2 months after surgery due to secondary malignancy—Squamous cell carcinoma, in his upper left eyelid.

without complications. In 2017 he developed "inflammation" of the right eye upper eye lid and was sent to an ophthalmologist for chalazion excochleation. By excisional biopsy was confirmed squamous cell carcinoma (**Figures 4** and **5**).

4. Conclusion

Retinoblastoma survivors as carriers of the retinoblastoma gene have a long life and increased incidence for secondary tumors. Ophthalmologists should always keep this in mind to be able to provide these patients with proper counseling, plan for close long-term follow-up, and update their knowledge in the therapy modalities of retinoblastoma current management and possible secondary malignancies in adulthood. A clear consensus on the form of a screening protocol would be most appropriate and effective in preventing future malignancies.

Conflict of interest

None of the authors has conflict of interest with this submission.

Printed form supported by KEGA 016 UK—4/2018 and APVV—17-0369.

Author details

Alena Furdova* and Juraj Sekac
Univerzita Komenského v Bratislave Lekárska fakulta Klinika oftalmológie LF UK Špitálska, Bratislava, Slovakia

*Address all correspondence to: alikafurdova@gmail.com

References

[1] Kamihara J, Bourdeaut F, Foulkes WD, Molenaar JJ, Mossé YP, Nakagawara A, et al. Retinoblastoma and neuroblastoma predisposition and surveillance. Clinical Cancer Research. 2017;**23**(13):e98-e106

[2] Fabian ID, Rosser E, Sagoo MS. Epidemiological and genetic considerations in retinoblastoma. Community Eye Health Journal. 2018; **31**(101):29-30

[3] Children's Oncology Group. Long-Term Follow-Up Guidelines for Survivors of Childhood, Adolescent, and Young Adult Cancers [Internet]. 2019. Available from: http://www.survivorshipguidelines.org/ [Accessed: January 8, 2019]

[4] Ellsworth RM. The practical management of retinoblastoma. Transactions of the American Ophthalmological Society. 1969;**67**: 462-534

[5] Nguyen HH, Nguyen HTT, Vu NP, Le QT, Pham CM, Huyen TT, et al. Mutational screening of germline RB1 gene in Vietnamese patients with retinoblastoma reveals three novel mutations. Molecular Vision. 2018;**24**: 231-238

[6] Shahraki K, Ahani A, Sharma P, Faranoush M, Bahoush G, Torktaz I, et al. Genetic screening in Iranian patients with retinoblastoma. Eye. 2017; **31**(4):620-627

[7] Molecular Study of Retinoblastoma in the Algerian Population. Screening of Rb gene in Constitutional and Tumoral Level. Semantic Scholar [Internet]. 2019. Available from: https://www.semanticscholar.org/paper/%5BMolecular-study-of-retinoblastoma-in-the-Algerian-Boubekeur-Louhibi/281deede31ab85275b31fa479a7804e25181bfbc [Accessed: January 9, 2019]

[8] Pendergrass TW, Davis S. Incidence of retinoblastoma in the United States. Archives of Ophthalmology. 1980;**98**(7): 1204-1210

[9] Broaddus E, Topham A, Singh AD. Survival with retinoblastoma in the USA: 1975–2004. The British Journal of Ophthalmology. 2009;**93**(1):24-27

[10] Kleinerman RA, Tucker MA, Abramson DH, Seddon JM, Tarone RE, Fraumeni JF. Risk of soft tissue sarcomas by individual subtype in survivors of hereditary retinoblastoma. Journal of the National Cancer Institute. 2007;**99**(1):24-31

[11] Aerts I, Pacquement H, Doz F, Mosseri V, Desjardins L, Sastre X, et al. Outcome of second malignancies after retinoblastoma: A retrospective analysis of 25 patients treated at the Institut curie. European Journal of Cancer. 2004;**40**(10):1522-1529

[12] Abramson DH, Frank CM. Second nonocular tumors in survivors of bilateral retinoblastoma: A possible age effect on radiation-related risk. Ophthalmology. 1998;**105**(4):573-579. Discussion 579-580

[13] Abramson DH, Melson MR, Dunkel IJ, Frank CM. Third (fourth and fifth) nonocular tumors in survivors of retinoblastoma. Ophthalmology. 2001; **108**(10):1868-1876

[14] Abramson DH, Fabius AWM, Francis JH, Marr BP, Dunkel IJ, Brodie SE, et al. Ophthalmic artery chemosurgery for eyes with advanced retinoblastoma. Ophthalmic Genetics. 2017;**38**(1):16-21

[15] Fletcher O, Easton D, Anderson K, Gilham C, Jay M, Peto J. Lifetime risks of common cancers among retinoblastoma survivors. Journal of the

National Cancer Institute. 2004;**96**(5):357-363

[16] Marees T, van Leeuwen FE, de Boer MR, Imhof SM, Ringens PJ, Moll AC. Cancer mortality in long-term survivors of retinoblastoma. European Journal of Cancer. 2009;**45**(18):3245-3253

[17] Marees T, van Leeuwen FE, Schaapveld M, Imhof SM, de Boer MR, Kors WA, et al. Risk of third malignancies and death after a second malignancy in retinoblastoma survivors. European Journal of Cancer. 2010;**46**(11):2052-2058

[18] Marees T, Moll AC, Imhof SM, de Boer MR, Ringens PJ, van Leeuwen FE. Risk of second malignancies in survivors of retinoblastoma: More than 40 years of follow-up. Journal of the National Cancer Institute. 2008;**100**(24):1771-1779

[19] MacCarthy A, Birch JM, Draper GJ, Hungerford JL, Kingston JE, Kroll ME, et al. Retinoblastoma in Great Britain 1963-2002. The British Journal of Ophthalmology. 2009;**93**(1):33-37

[20] Kleinerman RA, Yu C-L, Little MP, Li Y, Abramson D, Seddon J, et al. Variation of second cancer risk by family history of retinoblastoma among long-term survivors. Journal of Clinical Oncology: Official Journal of the American Society of Clinical Oncology. 2012;**30**(9):950-957

[21] Kleinerman RA, Schonfeld SJ, Tucker MA. Sarcomas in hereditary retinoblastoma. Clinical Sarcoma Research. 2012;**2**(1):15

[22] Wong JR, Morton LM, Tucker MA, Abramson DH, Seddon JM, Sampson JN, et al. Risk of subsequent malignant neoplasms in long-term hereditary retinoblastoma survivors after chemotherapy and radiotherapy. Journal of Clinical Oncology. 2014;**32**(29):3284-3290

[23] Schlienger P, Campana F, Vilcoq JR, Asselain B, Dendale R, Desjardins L, et al. Nonocular second primary tumors after retinoblastoma: Retrospective study of 111 patients treated by electron beam radiotherapy with or without TEM. American Journal of Clinical Oncology. 2004;**27**(4):411-419

[24] Newton WA, Meadows AT, Shimada H, Bunin GR, Vawter GF. Bone sarcomas as second malignant neoplasms following childhood cancer. Cancer. 1991;**67**(1):193-201

[25] Draper GJ, Sanders BM, Kingston JE. Second primary neoplasms in patients with retinoblastoma. British Journal of Cancer. 1986;**53**(5):661-671

[26] Hawkins MM, Wilson LM, Burton HS, Potok MH, Winter DL, Marsden HB, et al. Radiotherapy, alkylating agents, and risk of bone cancer after childhood cancer. Journal of the National Cancer Institute. 1996;**88**(5):270-278

[27] Hawkins BS, Collaborative Ocular Melanoma Study Group. The collaborative ocular melanoma study (COMS) randomized trial of pre-enucleation radiation of large choroidal melanoma: IV. Ten-year mortality findings and prognostic factors. COMS report number 24. American Journal of Ophthalmology. 2004;**138**(6):936-951

[28] Pillay R, Graham-Pole J, Novak L, Kurczynski E, Yulish BS. Successful treatment of osteogenic sarcoma developing as a second cancer in childhood. The American Journal of Pediatric Hematology/Oncology. 1983;**5**(1):103-105

[29] Turaka K, Shields CL, Meadows AT, Leahey A. Second malignant neoplasms following chemoreduction with carboplatin, etoposide, and vincristine in 245 patients with intraocular retinoblastoma. Pediatric Blood & Cancer. 2012;**59**(1):121-125

[30] Gombos DS, Hungerford J, Abramson DH, Kingston J, Chantada G, Dunkel IJ, et al. Secondary acute myelogenous leukemia in patients with retinoblastoma: Is chemotherapy a factor? Ophthalmology. 2007;**114**(7): 1378-1383

[31] Tucker MA, D'Angio GJ, Boice JD, Strong LC, Li FP, Stovall M, et al. Bone sarcomas linked to radiotherapy and chemotherapy in children. The New England Journal of Medicine. 1987; **317**(10):588-593

[32] Jenkinson HC, Winter DL, Marsden HB, Stovall MA, Stevens MCG, Stiller CA, et al. A study of soft tissue sarcomas after childhood cancer in Britain. British Journal of Cancer. 2007;**97**(5):695-699

[33] Moll AC, Imhof SM, Schouten-Van Meeteren AY, Kuik DJ, Hofman P, Boers M. Second primary tumors in hereditary retinoblastoma: A register-based study, 1945–1997: Is there an age effect on radiation-related risk? Ophthalmology. 2001;**108**(6):1109-1114

[34] MacCarthy A, Bayne AM, Brownbill PA, Bunch KJ, Diggens NL, Draper GJ, et al. Second and subsequent tumours among 1927 retinoblastoma patients diagnosed in Britain 1951–2004. British Journal of Cancer. 2013;**108**(12): 2455-2463

[35] Zhai Y-L, Nikaido T, Orii A, Horiuchi A, Toki T, Fujii S. Frequent occurrence of loss of heterozygosity among tumor suppressor genes in uterine leiomyosarcoma. Gynecologic Oncology. 1999;**75**(3):453-459

[36] Moore K, Tawfik O, Hays A, Opole I. Simultaneous low- and high-grade primary leiomyosarcomas in two separate organs in a thirty-year survivor of hereditary retinoblastoma. Case Reports in Oncological Medicine. 2015; **968567**:1-4

[37] de Jong MC, Kors WA, de Graaf P, Castelijns JA, Moll AC, Kivelä T. The incidence of trilateral retinoblastoma: A systematic review and meta-analysis. American Journal of Ophthalmology. 2015;**160**(6):1116-1126.e5

[38] Yamanaka R, Hayano A, Takashima Y. Trilateral retinoblastoma: A systematic review of 211 cases. Neurosurgical Review. 2019;**42**(1):39-48

[39] Wong FL, Boice JD, Abramson DH, Tarone RE, Kleinerman RA, Stovall M, et al. Cancer incidence after retinoblastoma. Radiation dose and sarcoma risk. The Journal of the American Medical Association. 1997; **278**(15):1262-1267

[40] Horowitz JM, Park SH, Bogenmann E, Cheng JC, Yandell DW, Kaye FJ, et al. Frequent inactivation of the retinoblastoma anti-oncogene is restricted to a subset of human tumor cells. Proceedings of the National Academy of Sciences of the United States of America. 1990;**87**(7):2775-2779

[41] Kleinerman RA, Tarone RE, Abramson DH, Seddon JM, Li FP, Tucker MA. Hereditary retinoblastoma and risk of lung cancer. Journal of the National Cancer Institute. 2000;**92**(24): 2037-2039

[42] Ştefănescu ML, Tomescu PI, Forţofoiu MC, Stoica LE, Badea O, Mogoanta L, et al. Urinary bladder tumors clinical and statistical retrospective study. Current Health Sciences Journal. 2018;**44**(1):64-70

[43] Mitra AP, Birkhahn M, Cote RJ. p53 and retinoblastoma pathways in bladder cancer. World Journal of Urology. 2007; **25**(6):563-571

[44] Kleinerman RA, Tucker MA, Tarone RE, Abramson DH, Seddon JM, Stovall M, et al. Risk of new cancers after radiotherapy in long-term survivors of retinoblastoma: An extended follow-up. Journal of Clinical Oncology: Official Journal of the

American Society of Clinical Oncology. 2005;**23**(10):2272-2279

[45] Sheppard KE, McArthur GA. The cell-cycle regulator CDK4: An emerging therapeutic target in melanoma. Clinical Cancer Research. 2013;**19**(19):5320-5328

[46] Travis LB, Ng AK, Allan JM, Pui C-H, Kennedy AR, Xu XG, et al. Second malignant neoplasms and cardiovascular disease following radiotherapy. Journal of the National Cancer Institute. 2012; **104**(5):357-370

[47] Henderson TO, Rajaraman P, Stovall M, Constine LS, Olive A, Smith SA, et al. Risk factors associated with secondary sarcomas in childhood cancer survivors: A report from the childhood cancer survivor study. International Journal of Radiation Oncology, Biology, Physics. 2012;**84**(1):224-230

[48] Leong SL, Chaiyakunapruk N, Lee SWH. Candidate Gene Association studies of anthracycline-induced cardiotoxicity: A systematic review and meta-analysis. Scientific Reports. 2017; 7(1):39

[49] Rodriguez-Galindo C, Wilson MW, Haik BG, Merchant TE, Billups CA, Shah N, et al. Treatment of intraocular retinoblastoma with vincristine and carboplatin. Journal of Clinical Oncology: Official Journal of the American Society of Clinical Oncology. 2003;**21**(10):2019-2025

[50] Mallipatna AC, Dimaras H, Chan HSL, Héon E, Gallie BL. Periocular topotecan for intraocular retinoblastoma. Archives of Ophthalmology. 2011;**129**(6):738-745

[51] Schouten-Van Meeteren AYN, Moll AC, Imhof SM, Veerman AJP. Overview: Chemotherapy for retinoblastoma: An expanding area of clinical research. Medical and Pediatric Oncology. 2002;**38**(6):428-438

[52] Chantada GL, Fandino AC, Carcaboso AM, Lagomarsino E, de Davila MTG, Guitter MR, et al. A phase I study of periocular topotecan in children with intraocular retinoblastoma. Investigative Ophthalmology & Visual Science. 2009; **50**(4):1492-1496

[53] Green DM, Nolan VG, Goodman PJ, Whitton JA, Srivastava D, Leisenring WM, et al. The cyclophosphamide equivalent dose as an approach for quantifying alkylating agent exposure. A report from the childhood cancer survivor study. Pediatric Blood & Cancer. 2014;**61**(1):53-67

[54] Foster MC, Kleinerman RA, Abramson DH, Seddon JM, Tarone RE, Tucker MA. Tobacco use in adult long-term survivors of retinoblastoma. Cancer Epidemiology, Biomarkers & Prevention. 2006;**15**(8):1464-1468

[55] Alkatan H, Maktabi A. Malignant fibrous histiocytoma in a patient with history of treated retinoblastoma. Saudi Journal of Ophthalmology. 2010;**24**: 23-26